T0151354

VINTAGE SECRETS

Hollywood

Diet and Fitness

Laura Slater

Plexus, London

Contents

Introduction

'You envy the glamour of the movie star that
you see in the movies. Well, so does Miss Movie Star.
She envies the glamorous image on the screen that
was once herself, and wishes she could be as
hotsy-totsy looking in real life.'

– Sylvia of Hollywood, diet and fitness guru of the 1920s and '30s

In the golden age of Hollywood glamour – before celebrities' least flattering photos were routinely splashed across tabloid papers and trashy magazines – motion picture actresses were visions of flawless beauty – goddesses of the silver screen. From Clara Bow to Joan Crawford, Rita Hayworth to Marilyn Monroe, these girls set the bar of beauty so high that the average woman could never hope to reach it. That didn't stop her trying, of course, and the growing diet industry was happy to help her.

This period saw the first widespread practice of crash dieting, the earliest commercial use of diet pills (and, later, appetite suppressants), the arrival of standardised clothing sizes in our stores, and diet foods on our supermarket shelves. It was in this era of Hollywood supremacy that the first celebrity diets – and celebrity diet gurus – began making an impact on the way ordinary women viewed their bodies.

Vintage Secrets: Hollywood Diet and Fitness looks at the diet and exercise fads of the 1920s-1950s, intended to turn office girls and housewives alike into movie star doubles; the methods the Hollywood beauties themselves employed to look their 'hotsy-totsy' best in real life;

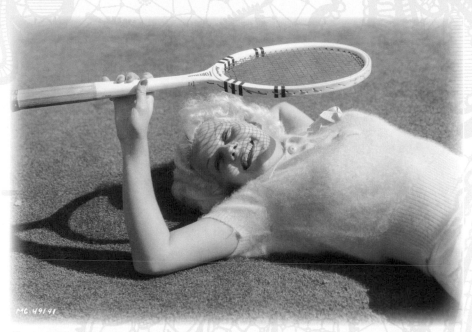

Above: Blonde beauty Jean Harlow believed in outdoor sports to boost circulation, enhance vitality and streamline the figure.

and the diet and fitness pros who helped them do it – much as today's star trainers help the rich and famous achieve their 'celebrity bodies'.

From those who, like Ava Gardner, ate to gain weight ('I have a diet that would put hips on a snake') to those who, like Jean Harlow, perpetually struggled to shed the pounds, this book takes a vintage look at our pursuit of the body beautiful. Exploring those fads, which (thankfully!) lost popularity, and those that (sometimes inexplicably) came back with a vengeance (cabbage soup diet, anyone?).

This is not a weight-loss manual: none of these diet and fitness routines are included as recommendations. These are merely illustrations of the various ways in which women have striven – more or less successfully – to conform to contemporary standards of beauty. From 1920s flappers, martyring themselves on the altar of slenderness, to the 'natural' beauties of the thirties, the health-conscious gals of the forties and the hourglass figures of the fifties, all have left their mark on the way we view food, dieting and our own bodies. Just as mothers influence their daughters, the women of the past have left a lasting legacy for the women of today.

Taking *the* Die Out *of* DIET

Hollywood, After Some Costly Experiments, Now Knows How To Reduce In Safety

By DOROTHY CALHOUN

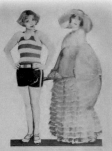

A recent visitor to Hollywood severely states that the natives have but two topics of conversation—the movies and bootleggers. Clive Brook remarks defensively that he has heard Hollywood gatherings discuss other subjects, among them dandruff! But there is one topic of unfailing interest and charm, suitable to any place, any company, both sexes, ever fresh, ever thrilling—and that is "diet." There is probably no place in the world where so many diet experiments are tried. In Hollywood, if you take care of the pounds, the pence will take care of themselves. The camera has a way of exaggerating size without mercy. One potato, recklessly indulged in, may cost a contract. "If I eat a chocolate cream, it shows in my next picture," moaned a film flapper recently. Almost all studios include a "weight clause" in their contracts. If the player passes the prescribed boundary, the contract is void. In succeeding issues of MOTION PICTURE we shall give our readers the benefit of the stars' experiences with successful and safe dieting, and publish menus, schedules and rules which have been tested and proved. In this article we point out some of the sad results, also learned by hard experience, of unscientific and unbalanced dieting in Hollywood.—Editor's Note

A RE the movie stars in earnest about their jobs?" said someone recently. "When a person is willing to go without food for a career, that person is in earnest. And half of the women—and men, too—in Hollywood deny themselves food. Most of the stars are hungry; only they call it by a more expensive name—dieting."

Two years ago Anna Q. Nilsson, then trium-

phantly carrying her blonde beauty from one important rôle to another in the movies, was thrown from her horse and broke her hip. The doctors promised that she would be about in three months at the latest. Several productions were postponed to await her recovery. But the broken bones did not knit as quickly as

they were expected to. Months passed in treatments, X-rays, diagnoses; the surgeons were frankly puzzled. Finally, they gathered for a consultation. They asked Anna for a full history of her case.

"Before I begin," she said, "perhaps I ought to tell you that I have practically starved myself for years . . ."

They listened, horrified, to her history of rigorous diets to which she had subjected her healthy Swedish appetite, for the sake of keeping a slender figure for the films. They heard of days of total fasting. And at the end they shook their heads gravely. "It is no wonder that your hip refused to heal properly," they said. "The wonder is that you are alive at all."

Eating to Live

A S they explained it," Anna says from the bed where she has undergone a recent and drastic operation, which it is believed will be successful, "I might have gone gaily along to the end of my days without any trouble from my wrong dieting—if this accident hadn't called upon my system suddenly for reserves of strength, and material for making new bone. And I had so depleted my reserves by years of careless dieting that there literally wasn't anything to repair the bone with. The lime and minerals I needed weren't there, that's all. Now I'm helping the operation with proper food and I'm going to walk as well as ever. But I've had two dreadful years—and I've learned my lesson! People simply can't get out of the habit of eating.

Acidosis, tuberculosis, heart failure, anemia —these are other bogeys waiting for the too adventurous dieter. And all these have had their victims in Hollywood. Stills from Greta Garbo's pictures made in

Sweden show a different girl, with plump arms, full bosom and what looks suspiciously like the beginnings of a double chin. The flat-chested, fleshless, almost haggard beauty of Greta Garbo to-day was purchased at the cost of months of strenuous and ill-balanced dieting which, it is admitted at the studio, brought on pernicious anemia and nearly made a lifelong invalid of one who had been a buxom young Swedish girl a few months before.

Diet Tragedies

B Y nature, Barbara La Marr was of the ripe, full-blown type of beauty, all soft curves and dimples. By movie code she was a vamp, and vampires, according to the specifications of the same code, were gaunt, sinuous creatures who wore slinky gowns. Plump ladies could not be imagined as harboring evil designs. So Barbara began to reduce, not wisely but too well. The gentle art of dieting was in its infancy in Hollywood at the time, and the few women who practised it more by strange combinations of food which were supposed to form a "thinning acid" in the stomach. One ate three meals a day of lamb chops and pineapple, or tomato and hard boiled eggs. Whatever it was that Barbara La Marr ate, or didn't eat, she soon sapped her reserves of strength so that her body could not respond to the terrific double strain of her screen work and her hectic private life. At thirty, with most of life before her, her beauty became haggard and tragic. Barbara La Marr died of tuberculosis, still crying gallantly to her friends, "Don't worry about me! I'll be living and making big money when I'm seventy."

Other victims of vanity and bad advice come to mind. There was Marietta Millner, imported from Germany by Paramount. In her native country they liked their women plump and femininely curved, but Ameri-

ca was different. Very well, if they wanted her thin, she would be thin! Again, it was a matter of self-starvation, of deliberately robbing her system of necessary elements. The result? A figure fleshless enough to satisfy American directors, and last year a grave, a very narrow grave, in a cemetery outside of Berlin. "Improper dieting," the papers said.

But against this list of stars on the black books of diet, there are a hundred others who have fought the good fight against flesh and have won—to the benefit of their looks and health. You might not think of Paul Whiteman as an example of successful re-

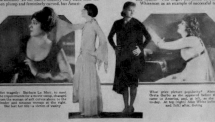

Diet tragedy: Barbara La Marr, to meet the requirements for a movie vamp, changed from the woman of soft curves above to the slender and sinuous woman at the right. She lost her life—a victim of vanity

What price picture popularity? Above, Greta Garbo as she appeared before she came to America, and, at left, as she is to-day. At top (right) Miss White before, and (left) after, dieting

---

Those Who Live Are The Ones Who Diet

ducing, but Paul (who weighed nineteen pounds at birth, and went right on from there) recently took off almost one hundred pounds in ten months. He weighed nearly three hundred pounds. He announces proudly that he is barely over two hundred now, and feels like another man. What did it? Massage? "Non-sense," sniffs Paul. Exercise? "Too much like work," grins Paul. It was diet, and nothing but diet, that did it—a sane diet of red meats and green vegetables and foods of low caloric content.

"Diet?" says Sylvia, the most famous masseuse in Hollywood, whose walls are decorated with hysterically grateful (and slim) photographs of the greatest stars of them all. "Diet is dangerous! They come to me after they have been dieting, with their glands so starved that their faces hang down and their necks are wrinkled, and their pores all enlarged with acidosis." But Sylvia, cornered, admits that she prescribes for her clients a "common sense menu" to accompany her massage. In the near future we hope to give you Sylvia's "common sense menu," which reads remarkably like a "diet."

Dozens of Daily Dozens

T HERE are a dozen expensive methods of reducing practised in Hollywood. There are massages,

and vapor baths, and strange machines that pound and roll the too, too solid flesh. There are all forms of exercise. There are other strange methods suggestive of the practices of Roman orgies—whispered about rather than proclaimed, by their devotees. Molly O'Day even had slices of fat carved from her legs, when the scales threatened to swing over the "weight limit" mentioned in her contract. The names of confirmed movie diet addicts are shown to a "reducing ring" in Hollywood, which floods them with folders and letters praising unheard methods of "Reduction by Thought Control," or "Weight Loss by Vibration," or enclosing samples of magic lotions "Guaranteed to Melt Fat Away." Louise Fazenda recently received a package of wafers through the mail, with a booklet promising an instant sylph-like figure. She laid them on a chair for a moment and her chow dogs ate them. "An hour later they were taken deathly sick and I sent them to the hospital," wails Louise. "I suppose they'll come back Dachshunds!"

(Continued on page 111)

Are You Sympathetic?

If you know what it means to keep at a certain weight—or very close to it—you will appreciate what it means to some of the well-known Hollywoodians listed below to keep within the weight limits prescribed for them.

How do they do it? Mostly by scientific diet. The list is full of surprises:

Player	Weight	Player	Weight
Richard Arlen	153	Dorothy Jordan	90
Jean Arthur	105	Helen Kane	119
George Bancroft	195	Dennis King	155
Clara Bow	108	Fred Kohler	200
Evelyn Brent	113	Gwen Lee	120
Mary Brian	110	Lila Lee	120
Clive Brook	119	Harold Lloyd	156
Nancy Carroll	116	Bessie Love	100
Ruth Chatterton	110	Jeanette MacDonald	110
Maurice Chevalier	160	Dorothy Mackaill	112
Bernice Claire	121	Jack Oakie	152
Gary Cooper	170	Catherine Dale Owen	125
Joan Crawford	115	Anita Page	119
Marion Davies	116	William Powell	178
Mary Doran	100	Charles Rogers	173
Kay Francis	112	Lillian Roth	118
Greta Garbo	125	Dorothy Sebastian	125
James Hall	158	Norma Shearer	114
Neil Hamilton	155	Raquel Torres	116
Hedda Hopper	125	Alice White	110
Leila Hyams	121	Fay Wray	102
Kay Johnson	122	Loretta Young	100

Contrasts: left tonight, below, Paul Whiteman, who took off nearly one hundred pounds by excellent dieting; Marietta Millner, who died from improper dieting; Anna Q. Nilsson, who now learns one must eat to live; and Molly O'Day, who reduced through surgery

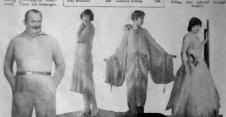

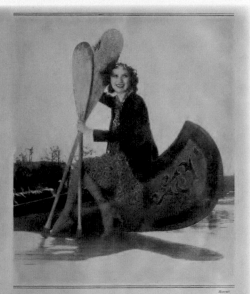

Hurrell

Can *oo'* Come Over

You often have heard of the river Jordan, and here she is, using her craft. And it's a short bet that Dorothy doesn't want to paddle her own canoe, or there wouldn't be two up with only one to go

* Spoken coquettishly, like the double o in Gama

1920s
Birth of the Modern Diet

'"Nobody loves a fat man" is a joke. "Nobody loves
a fat woman" is a tragedy, because in this day of the
"boyish" figure fixed by fashion as femininity's
final form, it is too, too often true.'

– Photoplay, 1924

Fitness gurus and fad diets, bobbed hair and bound breasts – welcome
to the 1920s. By the time the First World War was over, the curvy
Gibson Girl was but a distant memory as the ideal woman morphed
into a curiously androgynous figure. Plump was no longer pleasing. In
the fashion houses and on the silver screen, a new beauty standard was
being set – and the only curves allowed were concaves. Suddenly it was
a crime to be fat, and for the stars of the flourishing Hollywood studio
system, even more so – the camera *does* add ten pounds, after all.

Suburban housewives and silent screen sirens, New York socialites
and Parisienne fashion plates alike were tailoring their bodies to the
unforgiving lines of flapper fashions. Women became so *fashionably* thin
that they looked incapable of withstanding a stiff wind, let alone bearing
children. The press panicked and called it social rebellion. As much as
women going out to work, the barber's-pole figure was a challenge to
femininity. But in spite of press hysteria – and, for the most part, male
preferences – the 'fleshless look' persisted as the twenties ideal. So much

Opposite: **Motion Picture Magazine** *debates the pros and cons of dieting in one of
a series of melodramatic articles published throughout the 1920s and early '30s.*

7

so that by the early 1930s American women were several inches smaller – at all ages and across the board – than they had been a decade earlier.

Naturally, it was Hollywood – home of the glamorous and beautiful; land of outdoor, sun-dappled pursuits – that led the way in diet and exercise. The mere use of the word 'Hollywood' in an ad for fat-reducing soap or vibrating-belt treatments lent as much credibility to the product as the (often fictitious) doctor who created it. Stars were held up as shining examples of what a diet could do for *you*, little sister.

Even movie queens like Gloria Swanson were not ashamed to reveal the hard work that went into keeping slender for the super-sized screen. Looking attractive was a professional requirement and, almost as much

'There is probably no place in the world where so many diet experiments are tried. In Hollywood, if you take care of the pounds, the pence will take care of themselves.'

– Motion Picture Magazine, 1930

as the army of trainers, masseuses and dieticians who worked with them, movie stars were considered to be experts in physical culture. Hollywood diet and exercise routines appeared regularly in fan magazines for the benefit of would-be starlets, fuelling 1920s 'reduceomania' – and kicking off a trend for celebrity-endorsed diets that has never gone away.

The 1920s gave us calorie counting and bestselling diet books, a profusion of quick-fix 'reducing' regimes and a legion of perpetual dieters. Many twenties diets were unsound, to say the least. Designed to reduce women to wraith-like proportions, they put beauty firmly before health. A slender figure became a hallmark of success in life and love as women dieted in pursuit of an image, a lifestyle. For better or worse, the 1920s witnessed the birth of modern, aspirational dieting.

Opposite: Louise Brooks as the titular 'canary' in The Canary Murder Case *(1929). Brooks' slender, boyish figure made her a 1920s ideal.*

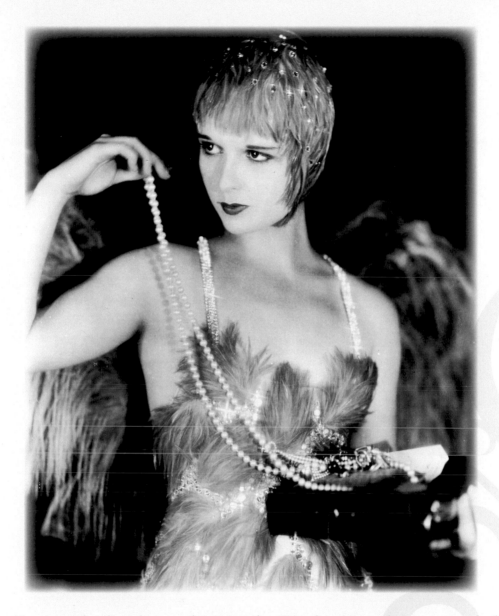

'I was asked to leave the Martha Washington, because people in a building overlooking the hotel had been shocked to see me on the roof, exercising in "flimsy pyjamas".'

– *Louise Brooks*

THE LAMB CHOP AND PINEAPPLE DIET

'These beauties of Hollywood and other
favoured cities who have adopted the Pineapple
and Lamb Chop Diet have done well.'

– Photoplay, 1924

One of the most popular twenties fads was the Lamb Chop and Pineapple plan. As the name suggests, this diet was about lamb chops and pineapple – and very little else. The theory was that lamb would give the dieter strength and pineapple would provide energy, while the acid in the pineapple would absorb any leftover fat from the (lean) lamb chops. In reality, like so many so-called 'magic pair' diets, the Lamb Chop and Pineapple plan really works by restricting your calories.

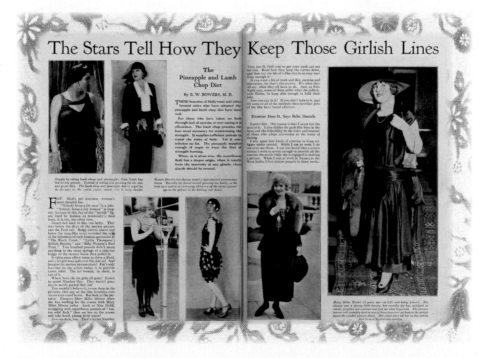

Above: Photoplay *reveals the stars' slimming secrets: everyone's eating lamb chops and pineapple.*

All the dieter has to do to achieve drastic weight loss is to put up with repetitive meals, hunger – and, naturally, a complete lack of carbohydrates – until he or she can no longer stand the sight of the 'magic' ingredients. Success depends on willpower – and the strength of your constitution.

A DAY ON THE LAMB CHOP AND PINEAPPLE PLAN

Breakfast: Two slices canned pineapple; two cups black coffee.

Lunch: One grilled lamb chop; one slice pineapple; one glass lemonade or iced tea.

Dinner: Two grilled lamb chops; two slices pineapple and a *demitasse*.

Silent screen vamp Nita Naldi, who lost twenty pounds in one month on the diet, had her own theory about the fashionable plan's rate of success: 'As nearly as I can tell, the Lamb Chop and Pineapple Diet cuts down your weight because it plays hob with the stomach,' she declared in a 1924 *Photoplay* article. Nita described the dieting experience as 'Hades'; she was literally starving herself, fainting in interviews – and still refusing to eat anything but her allotted portion of meat and tropical fruit. But, far from suggesting that the star might be overdoing it, the article saluted her dedication to the cult of slenderness. Anyone can look like a screen goddess was the message – but only if she is prepared to suffer.

Vintage Expert's Verdict: 'For those who have taken on flesh through lack of exercise or overeating [the diet] is efficacious. The lamb chop provides the lean meat necessary for maintaining the strength. It supplies sufficient protein to repair the waste of body. Yet it contributes no fat. The pineapple supplies enough of sugar to keep the fires of strength burning.' – EW Bowers, MD, 1924

Modern Expert's Verdict: 'Nutrition advances have taught us that eating a wide range of foods is the best way to lose weight. As always, if you want to shift those pounds safely and keep them off for good, you should never go below 1100 calories a day or follow an unbalanced diet that restricts the majority of foods while encouraging vast quantities of just a few.' – Dietician, Juliette Kellow BSc RD, 2011

THE GRAPEFRUIT DIET

'It was discovered that [the Hollywood Eighteen-Day Diet] was pretty dangerous medicine unless one had a strong constitution and was lolling on the sofa most of the time. However, it certainly gave the world a flock of sylphlike figures.'

– Grace Wilcox, The Milwaukee Journal, 1935

AKA: The (Hollywood) Eighteen-Day Diet, the Mayo Clinic Diet, the Protein and Citrus Diet . . .

The Grapefruit Diet was the hottest regime of the 1920s and, once again, it was based on 'magic' ingredients. Nobody really knows where the diet originated: some people credit the Mayo Clinic (which denies any involvement with the plan); some claim it was a clever marketing ploy from America's citrus growers; others say New York's elite restaurants cooked it up. Whatever the true story, it became an enormous twenties fad, spreading across the United States – and the Western world – like wildfire.

Advocates of the diet claimed that grapefruit contained a special enzyme with fat-burning properties. In reality, the plan, which permits just 585 calories a day, is a dangerous crash diet, one of many that became popular during the jazz era.

A DAY ON THE THE GRAPEFRUIT DIET

Breakfast: Half a grapefruit; one slice melba toast; tea or coffee

Lunch: Half a grapefruit; one hardboiled egg; six slices cucumber; one slice melba toast; tea or coffee.

Dinner: Half a grapefruit; two hardboiled eggs; half a lettuce; one tomato; tea or coffee

Banned foods included sugar, cream, salt or any seasoning.

Inevitably, the regime became associated with Hollywood, where screen sirens were rapidly redefining the shape of beauty. At A-list parties all over Tinseltown dinners would be served where no two guests – all on a different day of the regime – partook of the same meal. Studios reported money losses when their leading ladies collapsed from physical exhaustion (or nervous breakdowns), but the fad persisted until the 1930s. Many Los Angeles restaurants even adapted their menus to accommodate 'eighteen-dayers'.

Although doctors in the thirties declared the plan 'dangerous' – and, indeed a number of people are actually reported to have died from it – like so many fads, this one kept on coming back. Enjoying huge success in the 1980s, when the likes of Brooke Shields took up a marginally more generous 800-calorie version, the grapefruit regime was doing the rounds again in Hollywood as recently as 2004.

> 'Prominent among those losing weight through the Hollywood Diet are the apple growers of America. They lose five pounds every time they realise that they let citrus fruit men steal a march on them.'
>
> – HI Philips, Boston Globe, 1929

Vintage Expert's Opinion: 'In my series of articles on the Hollywood Diet, published a few weeks ago, I emphasised that these diets were dangerous because they offered less than half the food value that the average person needs to maintain strength and health and I said over and over that any too rapid reduction in weight is dangerous.' – Dr Morris Fishbein, Editor, *Journal of American Medical Association and Hygeia the Health Magazine*, 1929

Modern Expert's Opinion: 'Eating more grapefruit won't damage your health and can certainly contribute to a healthy diet.' However, the Grapefruit Diet is 'way too low in calories, extremely restrictive, unbalanced and, let's face it, incredibly boring!' – Dietician, Juliette Kellow BSc RD, 2011

THE FIRST DIET BESTSELLER

'You are in despair about being anything but fat,
and – ! how you hate it. But cheer up. I will save you;
yea, even as I have saved myself and many,
many others, so will I save you.'

– Dr Lulu Hunt Peters

It is simply *unpatriotic* to be fat in wartime. Just think, if people ate less they could send more food to the needy – or the troops. If they *spent* less on food, the money saved could benefit the Red Cross! Crucially, if fat people were just *thinner*, wouldn't they be more efficient, *useful* citizens? This is the gospel according to Dr Lulu Hunt Peters, author of *Diet and Health with a Key to the Calories*. For Dr Lulu, losing weight is not just about improving your own health; it's about improving the health of the nation. Perhaps this explains why her book, published while the First World War was still raging, became the world's first diet bestseller.

With the zeal of one who has already won the battle against unpatriotic pounds, the good doctor gets down to the business of helping her desperate readers to do the same. The method is simple and (in 1918) novel. They're going to think of food in terms of calories: 'Instead of saying one slice of bread, or a piece of pie, you will say 100 calories of bread, 350 calories of pie.' Dr Lulu doesn't much care *what* you eat – she cares how many calories you eat: ideally, fewer than you currently consume. If this means you gorge on 'luscious fat chocolates with curlicues on their tummies' and then resort to broth for dinner to balance things out – the doctor is okay with that. If you like a diet book that advocates skipping the meal and going straight to dessert, Dr Lulu might just have the plan for you!

In 1918, calories were still a new and somewhat controversial concept, so Dr Lulu takes some time to explain what they are and how they are calculated. Working out how many of these newfangled 'calories' you personally require to maintain your current weight – your 'maintenance diet' – involves even more maths. But once you've used your height, weight and (estimated) activity level to work out this magic number, all you have to do is eat less than this to achieve weight loss.

If you want to gain weight, of course, you need to eat *over* your maintenance diet. But then who wants to *gain* weight?

> 'How anyone can want to be anything but thin is beyond my intelligence.'
>
> *– Dr Lulu Hunt Peters*

FINDING YOUR IDEAL WEIGHT

Multiply number of inches over 5' in height by 5½; add 110. For example: Height 5' 7" without shoes.

7 x 5½ =	38½
	+ 110
	———
Ideal weight	148½ lbs

If under 5' multiply number of inches under 5' by 5½ and subtract from 110.

FINDING THE NUMBER OF CALORIES NEEDED

1. Determine normal weight by rule.

2. Multiply normal weight by number of calories needed per pound per day.

PER POUND PER DAY

Infants require	40-50 C.
Growing children require	30-40 C.
Adults (depending upon activity) require	15-20 C.
Old age requires	15 or less C.

Now, if you want to lose, cut down 500-1000 calories per day from that.

Clara Bow's

SUMMER DIET

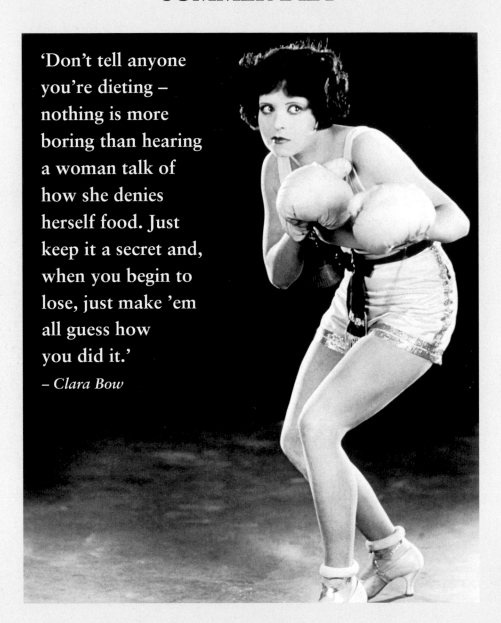

'Don't tell anyone you're dieting – nothing is more boring than hearing a woman talk of how she denies herself food. Just keep it a secret and, when you begin to lose, just make 'em all guess how you did it.'

– *Clara Bow*

You don't become Hollywood's original 'It' girl without making some sacrifices. For fickle fame, Clara Bow swallowed her pride and abandoned her privacy; she also gave up eating what she liked. Yet try as she might, Clara always had a fatal 'tendency to curves'. Clara arrived in Tinseltown as a hot little jazz baby aged just seventeen. Though she was required to lose weight for the screen – who wasn't? – Clara's irrepressible curves were largely tolerated for the sake of her undeniable sex appeal. But when she passed plump the studio drew the line. By the time she hit 23 (and 130 lbs), Clara's costumes were starting to arrive with a girdle and the executives at FOX threatened to exploit the weight clause in her contract. Curves, within limits, were permissible: double chins were not.

'Did you know that eating is one of the things Clara Bow is fondest of? When she's away from Hollywood, she doesn't miss boyfriends, but her cook! Maybe this explains some of Clara's curve-trouble in the past!'

– *Photoplay, 1931*

A desperate Clara repeatedly relied on dangerous crash diets to keep under the threshold of 118 lbs: the weight at which the studio could cancel her contract at ten days' notice. Although, like many stars, her household staff included an excellent cook, the meals this gastronome whipped up were rather grim: 'grapefruit juice and coffee for breakfast; an egg, a tomato and toast, and tea for lunch; and a lamb chop or steak, tomato and coffee for dinner.' The calorie total must have been somewhere in the region of 500 – hardly enough to keep a girl going during a long day on set.

A TYPICAL MENU FOR CLARA BOW

Breakfast: One large glass of orange juice.

Lunch: A crisp salad without mayonnaise; a leafy vegetable; toast; tea or coffee without cream.

Four O'Clock Tea: A cooling lemonade or other fruit drink.

Dinner: As meatless as possible. Pork and beef are absolutely banned. Favourite items included lamb chops, fish, vegetables, salads, cheese, cold consommés and toast.

CLARA'S EXERCISE ROUTINE

'I'd roll around the room like a rubber
ball until I was so dizzy that I couldn't move.
Then I'd jump up and stagger to the looking glass to
see if I'd lost any fat . . . Say, I'll bet I rolled a hundred
miles in that little room. I must be the champion roller
of the world. And I starved myself, too. But it worked.
Everybody noticed that I was getting thinner.'

– Photoplay, June 1925

In addition to her depressing diet, Clara made use of her 'big, well-equipped gymnasium' and, like many in sunny Hollywood, she also pursued outdoor sports in order to 'preserve the girlish figure that the public demands of its picture heroines'. According to one article in a fan magazine, Clara rode every morning and played tennis every evening. She also hiked and swam. But for rapid weight reduction, Clara was a firm believer in the popular twenties fat-reducing method of rolling around on the floor. Apparently, rolling on a hard surface would crush the fat off your body – especially if you wore tight clothing to prevent the flesh spreading out laterally.

In a 1922 article in *Motion Picture Magazine*, would-be screen actress (and wife of the editor) Corliss Palmer explains the 'science' of rolling off your fat:

> 'Rolling should be done on the floor. The hard surface does not yield to the contour of the body as the bed does, but resists and by its resistance crushes the cells of fat. A tight fitting, inelastic garment should be worn as it holds the flesh compactly, keeping it from yielding to the floor in any direction by spreading out laterally. This causes greater

weight and pressure on the flesh and therefore is more effective in crushing the cells of fat.

'Do not roll in a relaxed condition. Tighten up the muscles from head to toe. Keep your arms pressed close to your side. Start the rolling motion with the shoulders and heels. Roll as far in one direction as the space will permit. Now roll back in the opposite direction. Since you must not use your arms or your knees, you will find that every muscle in your body is required to keep rolling. Three minutes of this the first day is quite enough, and may be increased slowly or rapidly after that, according to the effect of the nerves and muscles. It will undoubtedly cause soreness at first, which may be remedied by the hot bath before retiring.'

Clara's Top Exercise Tip: 'Drink a cup of tea and eat a soda cracker just after [exercising]. This takes away the keenness of the appetite and makes it possible to eat moderately – to pass by the potatoes and pastry without cringing.'

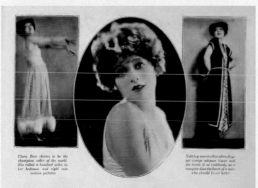

Clara Bow claims to be the champion roller of the world. She rolled a hundred miles in her bedroom and right into motion pictures

Nothing worries this ultra-flapper except adipose tissue and she treats it so ruthlessly as a vampire does the heart of a man who should know better

She Rolls Her Own—Fat Away

This is the story of a fat little school girl— who rolled across the bedroom floor to fame

By Glenn Chaffin

PHYSICIANS say that if her heart had been weak she'd be an angel now. But her heart was strong—and now she's a picture actress.

It is the story of how Clara Bow, recorded in the legends of Hollywood as an ultra-flapper, beat the Brooklyn department stores out of another tubby ribbon clerk and gave to Hollywood a rollicking gaiety that has stirred the pulse of its languid social realm.

Three years ago this little girl, who has journeyed with incredible swiftness along the trail of film achievement during the last year and a half, was studying ancient history in a Brooklyn high school and writing letters to the Answer Man of PHOTOPLAY.

She was fatter than most of her chums, but that didn't worry her. Nothing worried her. Her eyes were big and brown and filled with wonder. Filled with the wonder of youth, with the wonder of life that she knew little of and worried not at all about.

She wasn't even a flapper yet. But since that time she has given this nation of staccato standards its most vivid conception of this fantastic classification of girlhood and declares earnestly that she has bidded her flapper wings and is undertaking the serious business of being a grown up young lady.

Until a year ago, when she was selected one of the thirteen "Baby Stars" of the Wampas (Western Motion Picture Advertisers) annual frolic, I had never heard of Clara Bow. So obscure are the early rounds of the ladder of motion picture recognition.

Since that time I have seen her often, here and there along the boulevard which is Hollywood's "Main Street," and on studio sets where I have watched her work.

A short time ago in her bungalow home, which is located on the western residential end of that street, she told me the story of the fat little girl who threw her ancient history at a school chum who told her that she was too fat to be a film actress, and joined the ranks of those who figure in the columns of the Answer Man.

"I read a story in a newspaper about a beauty contest which offered as a prize a part in a motion picture," she said.

"I had just had my picture taken and decided that I was pretty. That was easy, for every girl who isn't pug-nosed thinks she's pretty.

"Daddy and I took a trolley over to the building where the contest was being held. What a shock I got. There were limousines lined up in front of the place and parked clear around the block. I saw a dozen girls enter the building and they all looked beautiful to me. I wanted to go back home right there but Daddy said, 'Come on. We'll give it a whirl, anyway.'

"Well, sir, the judges must have all been near sighted. Will you believe it? I was the prize."

I looked at the fascinating little youngster, curled with lazy grace in the great hollow of an upholstered rocking chair, and believed. There, with the warm light of a rose-shaded floor lamp softing the redness of her hair, its mellow glow blending with the vivid brown of her eyes, I would have believed her had she told me that she was Mona Lisa. [CONTINUED ON PAGE 113]

78

[CONTINUED ON PAGE 113]

'CLARA BOW is more than just a movie star. She is the living symbol of the Modern Girl. Her name is synonymous with jazz and Flaming Youth. She is the goddess of the new freedom. No star since the days of Valentino has had such a wide influence on the manners, clothes and behaviour of a devoted public.'

– Photoplay, August 1928

CLEAN EATING WITH
Gloria Swanson

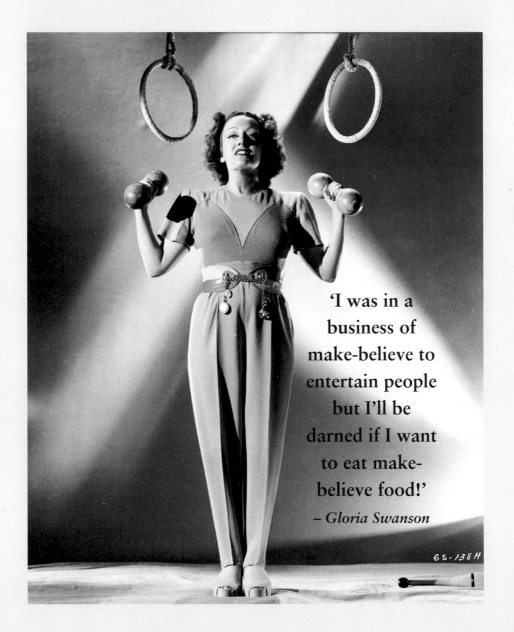

'I was in a business of make-believe to entertain people but I'll be darned if I want to eat make-believe food!'
– *Gloria Swanson*

GS-138H

Perhaps Hollywood's first Diva, at the height of her screen career Gloria Swanson was the image of the hedonistic twenties. Then the highest-paid woman in movies, she lived – and ate – in appropriately lavish fashion. She regularly indulged in six-course dinners with 'fish, meat, fancy sauces, hot breads, wine, rich desserts as well as cocktail sandwiches first'. To compensate for her decadent lifestyle, she would diet periodically with the help of Pathé's nutrition expert, a formidable little Norwegian known as Madame Sylvia.

But in 1928, while making her final silent film, the unfinished fiasco *Queen Kelly*, Gloria fell ill. Rather than doling out pills, her doctor asked her to describe what she had eaten in the past 24 hours. It was a revelation. Overnight, Gloria completely changed the way she ate, becoming a vegetarian and an outspoken advocate for raw foods and health foods. Soon she was making her own flour from brown rice, boiling organic raisins to make 'sugar' and arriving at fancy hotels, toting organic vegetables and a pressure cooker.

AN AVERAGE DAY ON THE GLORIA SWANSON DIET

Breakfast: Irish seaweed extraction, cooked in distilled water to avoid the chemicals in tap water.

Lunch: Cottage cheese, yellow peaches and water cress; 'Swedish type' crackers and butter.

Dinner: Chard and string beans (always yellow variety), pressure cooked without salt. Fish if 'I can see it caught with my own eyes'. Organic fruit, especially grapefruit, papayas, melon, or bananas – she liked it 'untampered with'.

Long before the clean eating craze, Gloria Swanson spoke out against unseen killers in the American diet, from sugar and 'bleached' flour to pesticides and preservatives. Most of her contemporaries thought her diet was crazy but she ignored them – wisely, as it turns out! As she continued to expound on her favourite theme – and to defy the ageing process – the world began to accept that the 'eccentric' star might have the right idea after all.

'Mary Duncan was a picture of woe . . .
From an average point of view, there was nothing
at all the matter with the girl. But the camera's
is not the average point of view'
– *Hollywood Undressed by Sylvia Ullback*

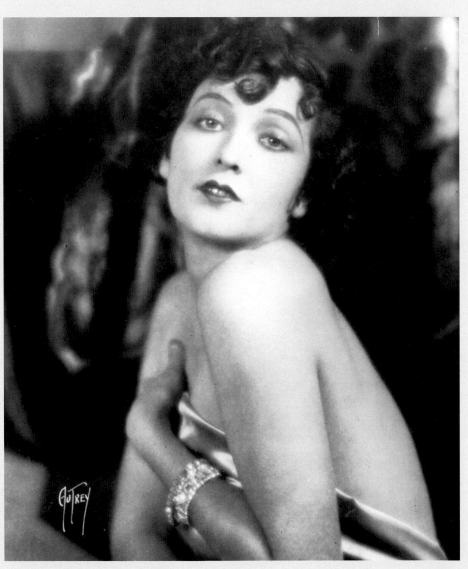

Madame Sylvia

HOLLYWOOD'S FIRST FITNESS GURU

'Sylvia Ullback, masseuse extraordinaire of Hollywood,
the flesh sculptor who pounds, beats and
curses the stars into shape.'

– Photoplay, 1931

Between 1926 and 1932, Sylvia Ullback – aka Madame Sylvia of Hollywood – was the woman Tinseltown turned to when its stars were suffering from 'avoirdupois'. Her clientele was a who's who of Hollywood's elite, including Gloria Swanson, Mary Pickford, Carole Lombard and Jean Harlow.

Sylvia extolled the virtues of diet, exercise and massage but her methods – which included techniques for swatting and squeezing off fat – would certainly raise a few eyebrows in Los Angeles today. Actresses apparently lined up to experience this brutal treatment because of Sylvia's suspect belief that, during a beating, 'the fat comes out of the pores like mashed potato through a colander'. During the course of her energetic work, she claimed to have stripped exactly 9,037 ½ pounds off of Hollywood's collective waistline.

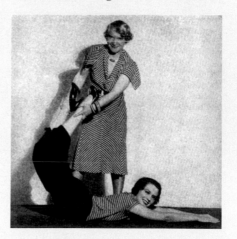

'One cannot be beautiful until one is well nourished.'

– Madame Sylvia

HOW SYLVIA WHIPPED
CAROLE INTO SHAPE

When Pathé decided to make a leading lady out of curvy Carole Lombard, they called in Madame Sylvia to effect the transformation. Sylvia recommended a strict diet, stretching and swaying exercises and, naturally, massage. Poor Carole was subjected to 'pounding, squeezing, pulling and pinching' and, according to Sylvia, she enjoyed it: 'Carole used to jump up from my treating table and dance around like a kid just because she felt so good!' the masseuse claimed.

Carole was apparently the perfect 'patient', uncomplainingly sticking to Sylvia's Spartan meal plan, and painful exercises. She had her reward: the diet worked, reducing Carole from a then-US size sixteen (approx. 28" waist) to a size twelve (approx. 25" waist). What's more, once she'd lost the weight, Carole never had to diet again. She used her common sense to keep thin, avoiding unhealthy food but generally eating what she liked in moderation.

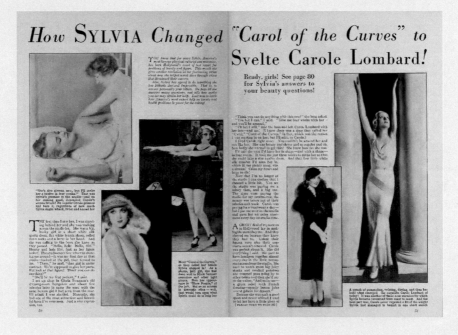

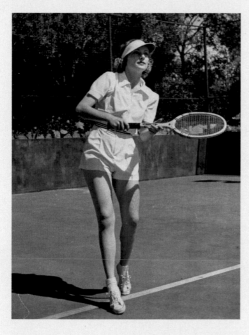

'How did I reduce Carole Lombard from a sixteen to a twelve? I'll tell you. For two hours every day I pounded and squeezed and slapped that flesh away.'

– *Madame Sylvia*

SYLVIA'S DIET FOR CAROLE LOMBARD

Although it contained whole grains and protein to fill her up in the morning, plenty of fruit and vegetables, and even occasional treats, Sylvia's diet for Carole is certainly Spartan. According to Sylvia, the diet contained plenty of food that would 'produce red blood', preventing anaemia.

Breakfast: Small glass orange juice; small glass water; one slice whole wheat toast with a smear of butter; coddled egg; black coffee.

Lunch: Glass tomato juice; half a head of lettuce; one sliced tomato and French dressing (mostly lemon juice). Dish of gelatin with spoonful of thin coffee cream. Iced tea.

Mid-Afternoon Snack: Tomato or orange juice.

Dinner: Small bunch of celery; two lamb chops; baked potato skin.

Treat: A small piece of angel food cake with a large glass of iced tea.

EARLY COSMETIC SURGERY

In the 1920s, 'sweat and slap' gurus like Sylvia did a roaring trade. But if you think Sylvia's treatments sound bad, you should spare a thought for the silver screen stars who subjected themselves to far more drastic forms of fat removal. The 1920s saw some of the earliest attempts at liposuction. Of course, many Hollywood actresses were just desperate enough to try it.

In the best-case scenario, the doctor would surgically remove the fat with a scalpel. If this wasn't particularly effective, nor was it especially dangerous. A second popular method was to melt fat away with electric needles – the process could take several excruciating hours to complete. It was to this second, hideous method that budding screen actress Molly O'Day turned in pursuit of stardom.

Identified as a promising actress by First National, Molly signed to the studio on the understanding that she would have to 'reduce' if she wanted to work as a leading lady. Initially, Molly did lose weight with the help of a studio-assigned dietician. Once left to her own devices, however, the pounds soon piled back on so that, as one producer phrased it, she became 'pathetically fleshy'.

Molly's weight was not just an affront to her producer's aesthetic sensibilities, however; her extra poundage actually put her career in jeopardy. Pretty and talented as she was, her rosy apple cheeks and healthy plumpness constituted a violation of the 'facial and physical disfigurement' clause in her contract; the studio were within their rights to drop the young actress if she didn't shape up. Unable to stick to the depressing diets assigned to her by the studio dieticians or to mould her figure to leading-lady lines by any other method, Molly went under the surgeon's knife. The results were not happy.

Opposite: 'Baby star' Molly O'Day was one of many actresses who resorted to the surgeon's knife when she reached the infamous 'weight limit' in her contract.

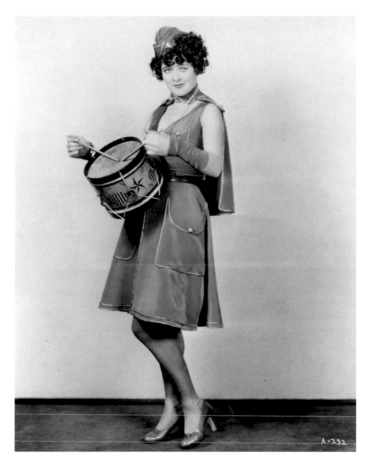

'It was while she was on location for *Little Shepherd of Kingdom Come* that she began her dissipation, friends tell us. Not in the day time. Oh, no! For there was the dietician always ready with spinach and lamb chops and pineapple. But at night, on the sly, like a school kid . . . Twenty pounds – well, twenty pounds is enough to ruin even a long-established, ultra-well known, motion-picture lady.'

– *Photoplay, August 1928*

RAW

'Now, what is raw food exactly?'
'Vegan non-dairy. And nothing is cooked over 118 degrees.'
'In other words, raw vegetables.'
'And sometimes flowers.'

Sex and the City, Season 6, Episode 2, 'Great Sexpectations', 2003

Back in 2003, when the girls from *Sex and the City* set out to sample the lukewarm delicacies offered by New York's hottest new restaurant, Raw, the raw food movement was just the latest celebrity fad. Madonna, Demi Moore, Alicia Silverstone – the list of beautiful people advocating the health benefits of raw food was getting longer by the minute. But, for most of us, the idea of giving up cooked meals forever was a bit of a joke. The restaurant that features in the episode isn't even real.

Then, all of a sudden, raw food went mainstream, and it wasn't just New York socialites and LA hippies who were chowing down on pulses whilst knocking back a wheatgrass shot. Raw food restaurants even began popping up in such unlikely places as Yorkshire, spiritual home of the roast dinner. Today, a raw food diet is just another lifestyle choice, hardly more surprising than veganism.

> **'This diet is time-consuming, socially isolating and you'll have an awful lot of chewing to do.'**
>
> *– The British Dietetic Association*

Followers of the raw food diet do seem to lose weight – the restricted food selection means the diet is usually lower in calories – and many claim they feel and look younger and more vibrant. But it has yet to be scientifically proven that excluding *all* cooked foods is the way to go. While some nutrients in food are undoubtedly destroyed by cooking, others cannot be absorbed if the food is eaten raw. And, of course, if you aren't going to cook anything there is a wide range of food that is unwise or unsafe to eat. Try raw potato and you're likely to get a stomach ache; try raw chicken and you could get a lot worse!

The subject is still controversial – newspapers and magazines never seem to get tired of talking about raw food – but if you thought the debate only started a decade ago, think again: the movement has its roots in European Naturalist philosophies of the late 19th century and, by the 1920s, it had outspoken advocates in sunny California, where it was being toted as a cure for everything from migraines to cancer.

> ## '[The Natural Food System] gets results – not only the negative results of freedom from sickness and fatigue, but creates a new feeling of well-being and vigor.'
>
> *– Mrs Richter's Cook-Less Book*

Vera and John Richter opened America's first raw food restaurant in Los Angeles in 1917. The Eutropheon (Greek for 'good nourishment') catered to the health-conscious and idly curious for over 25 years. Mr Richter gave regular lectures on 'natural living' and, in 1922, *Mrs Richter's Cook-Less Book* enabled rawfoodists to recreate the restaurant's dishes at home.

Although no famous stars were known to go entirely raw, some, like Greta Garbo, consciously explored the idea, and others, like Lillian Gish, ate a partially raw diet because they enjoyed the taste (her favourite combination was carrot and apple salad).

VINTAGE INSPIRATION
VERA RICHTER'S COW-LESS ICE CREAM

2 lbs ripe bananas, macerated
2 lbs strawberries, macerated
1 lb honey
1 lb pinenuts (or peanuts), flaked
2 pints water

Combine well and freeze.

This recipe is high fibre, low sodium, vegetarian and raw.

Greta Garbo

FITNESS FANATIC

'Beauty is a matter of health.'

– *Greta Garbo*

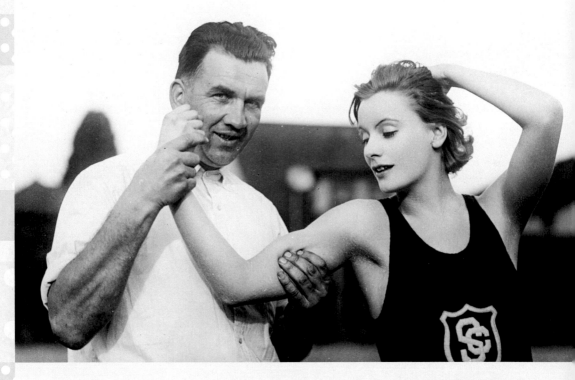

'Having known Dr Bieler for some years, I am sure that his
book *Food is Your Best Medicine*, will be a great help
for many people in their fight against disease.'

– *Greta Garbo*

It's easy to forget that 'the face of the century' also possessed an elegant figure. Greta Garbo made a career out of languid gestures, but off-screen she put time and energy into living well. She practiced an array of sports, always kept abreast of the latest fitness trends, and took real pleasure from munching on a raw vegetable salad.

Although The Great Garbo was famously made to lose weight – twice – to make it into Hollywood movies, she does seem to have held a genuine interest in eating – and living – well. She made a conscious effort to keep herself in tip-top condition and a recent auction of personal belongings from her estate provides ample evidence of her active lifestyle and long-time interest in health and fitness. Yoga outfits, walking shoes, dance slippers, ski gear, swimming costumes, tennis rackets, a juicer, medicine balls and an array of health and fitness books were all to be found in her New York apartment.

In the 1940s, Greta famously became a student and close friend of Hollywood diet guru Gayelord Hauser, but her interest in diet and fitness began before – and went beyond – his teachings. Although Greta's shelves were crowded with books on diet and health, Dr Henry Bieler's *Food is Your Best Medicine* is the only book the elusive star ever endorsed.

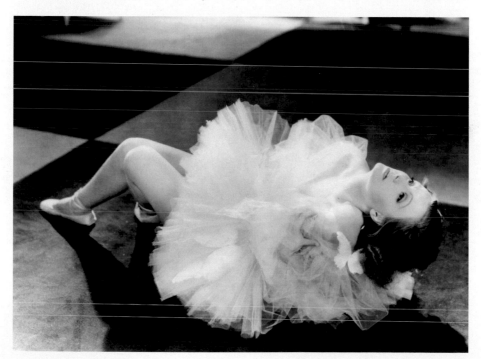

Dr Henry Bieler

PUSHING THE BOUNDARIES OF (ALTERNATIVE) MEDICINE

'Dr Bieler taught me in 1927 that your body is the direct result of what you eat as well as what you don't eat. Every day I live merely reinforces his lessons.'

– *Gloria Swanson*

Dr Henry Bieler was Hollywood's go-to diet man decades before his bestselling book, 1965's *Food is Your Best Medicine*, made him a household name. In the 1920s, Mary Pickford, Gloria Swanson and Greta Garbo were just three of the many famous clients who swore by his simple principles: stop popping pills and start eating well instead.

Dr Bieler taught that most illnesses were caused by the build-up of toxins in the body – and that this *toxemia* was the direct result of eating the wrong things. It followed, therefore, that eating the *right* foods could prevent diseases; from arthritis, heart disease and tumours, to migraines, nervousness, skin diseases and obesity, as well as hosts of minor ailments like coughs, colds and allergies, all of these might be avoided simply by eating better.

'The patient I am treating must be exhaustively studied, his condition recognised. If possible, he must be relieved of his symptoms and cured. That is why this book must remain general. It is not a recipe for getting well.'

– *Dr Henry Bieler, Food is Your Best Medicine*

Recognising that we are all individuals, Bieler refused to prescribe a 'cure-all diet'. Instead, he put forward general principles for healthy eating. Well ahead of his time, he recommended whole, organic foods and, where

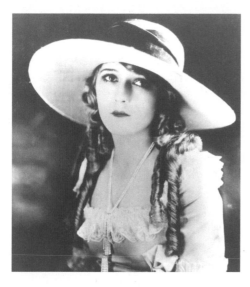

'Overindulgence in eating causes an ugly complexion, which mocks you from the screen. Too many sweets ruin the teeth, affect the digestion, injure the eyes and have a disastrous effect upon the hair.'

– Bieler follower, Mary Pickford

possible, *raw* foods – this included raw eggs and very rare beef and lamb. He preferred digestible proteins like raw goats' milk to cows' milk. And his banned list included starches, additives, preservatives, pasteurised milk, cooked egg whites and stimulants such as sugar, salt and caffeine.

Unlike many faddish diets of the twenties, Dr Bieler warned his followers not to expect instantaneous results. His diet was part of a lifestyle change and he cautioned that ridding yourself of habits – and your body of toxins – takes time. What's more, Dr Bieler recognised that sticking to a healthy diet is not always as easy as it sounds – especially if, like many of his star clients, you have a busy life. 'Sometimes the patient, unlike the horse, knows the life-saving water is there, but his professional life is so arranged that he cannot (or so he believes) stick to his therapeutic diet,' Bieler conceded.

'Even one correct meal aids a toxin-saturated body.'

– Dr Henry Bieler

Although his stance against surgery and traditional medicines outraged many of his contemporaries, the past half-century has confirmed many of Dr Bieler's teachings: food choices *do* have a huge impact on overall health – reports from the American Medical Association suggest 70 percent of health problems might be avoided by better nutrition. *Food is Your Best Medicine* (1965) is still in print and regarded as a nutrition classic.

1930s
Health, Vitality and Personality!

'Be a Garbo if you must, but be a Harlow if you can!'
– Motion Picture, March 1932

The 1930s saw a move away from the boyish look, with womanly curves making a modest comeback. But just because women were permitted to look like, well, *women*, that didn't halt the progress of the diet bug – far from it! Only the emphasis had shifted. In inter-war Europe and Depression-era America, hardship and increased awareness of health and nutrition brought with them a new kind of dieting, based (in theory, at least) on common sense. On the screen and on the street, the watch words of the 1930s were 'health', 'vitality' and 'personality'.

Where the 1920s had been an era of excess, the 1930s saw the return of moderation – in terms of dieting this meant striving for a 'natural look' after the 'artificial' thinness of the previous decade. According to Florenz Ziegfeld (he of Broadway's *Ziegfeld Follies*), the perfect 1930s woman had a 'softly feminine contour' – not the sharp angles of the flapper girl. Nobody wanted to be rail-thin anymore. The likes of Greta Garbo – previously untouchable – began attracting criticism as the press made dark allusions to diet-induced health problems.

1920s Hollywood had gained a reputation for freedom, equality – and moral laxity. The town was beset by scandal, and many people found it hard to distinguish between the steamy storylines and risqué characters of the screen and the actors and actresses who starred in such 'immoral' films. With the papers spinning lurid tales of debauchery and excess, stars

> ## 'Curves mean health, and health means vitality and verve – these things create personality.'
> ### – *Florenz Ziegfeld*

had been determined to show that they worked pretty damn hard, thank you very much. They cited their vigorous fitness regimens in response to those who said theirs was a life of luxury and (over)indulgence.

But, by the 1930s, Hollywood had suffered the double-blow of censorship and the Great Depression. On-screen and off, lifestyles were more subdued and the message coming out of movieland was one of restraint. Although most stars did still diet – and some of them even admitted to it – it was far more fashionable to be naturally and effortlessly young and beautiful. Everybody wanted to be healthy, clean and wholesome: a Ginger Rogers type.

Advertising and popular magazines took the same tone, promoting health and nutrition even as they surreptitiously suggested that a fat girl would end life unloved and alone. Health and fitness columns in publications such as France's *Votre Santé* and the British *Lady's Companion* continued to publish 'scientific'

> ## 'Last year it was the 18-day diet. This year it is "eat and exercise".'
> ### – *The Boston Globe, July 5, 1931*

reducing regimes; ads for reducing aids, corsetry and diet pills proliferated in Hollywood fan magazines and newspapers alike. All promoted a womanly figure, albeit a very slender one. It was around this time that WK Kellogg made a hit with his nutritious All-Bran cereal, designed to help you 'Keep Healthy While You Are Dieting to Reduce!' Of course, the campaign had Hollywood endorsement.

If anything, the diet craze gained momentum in the 1930s and, while the very thin were branded fanatics, in such difficult times, the overweight were considered just plain greedy. *Over*-dieting was certainly frowned upon, but to be fat when so many were struggling to put food on the table was criminal. And of course, extra weight remained aesthetically displeasing; cosmetics magnate Helena Rubinstein was certainly not alone in thinking fat was 'something repulsive'. Bombarded, as we are today, with conflicting messages – cautions against crash diets; warnings that being overweight could only lead to misery – the 1930s girl had a decision to make: to diet or not to diet? To diet, of course.

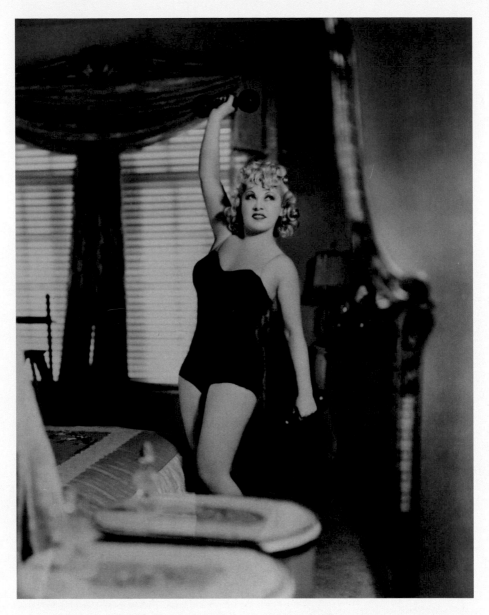

'Cultivate your curves – they may be dangerous but they won't be avoided.'

– *Mae West*

FORGET DIET AND EXERCISE
(TRY PILLS AND CIGARETTES)

'Dorothy [Gish] dieted with no effect,
and would you believe it she took up smoking and
lost pounds with no ill effects and now she's better
pleased with her weight and perfectly healthy.'
– *Lillian Gish, The Pittsburgh Post-Gazette, Nov 29, 1929*

The 1930s saw a boom in metabolism-boosting wonder drugs – the prevailing theory being that a sluggish metabolism was at the root of most obesity problems. First developed for commercial use in Germany in the 1880s, pills containing thyroid extract – to stimulate underperforming glands – soon spread beyond Europe and had arrived in the US by 1908.

By 1935, 100,000 Americans had tried the drugs, which promised quick slimming without the need for diet or exercise. Dinitrophenol – a dying agent used in explosives and pesticides – was the most popular ingredient in these pills, which made dieters hot and sweaty as their metabolism increased. Apparently, one could lose one or two pounds a week by taking the pills without any change to diet. Unfortunately, the sweats were the least of dinitrophenol's many side effects, which also included rashes, damage to sense of taste and eye cataracts, as well as, occasionally, liver failure and death. By 1938, the drug had been pulled from the market.

For those who preferred to avoid pills, another dieter's friend – with its own, not so obvious, health risks – was the good old cigarette. In the early thirties, popular brand Lucky Strike began targeting women with the slogan 'Reach for a Lucky instead of a sweet'. The idea caught on: more than one silver screen goddess claimed smoking kept her slim. Today, despite increased awareness of the dangers of cigarettes, many women still employ them as a diet aid.

THE HAY DIET

'Any carbohydrate foods require alkaline conditions for their complete digestion, so must not be combined with acids of any kind, such as sour fruits, because the acid will neutralise. Neither should these be combined with a protein of a concentrated sort as these protein foods will excite too much hydrochloric acid during their stomach digestion.'

– William Hay, How to Always Be Well

Smoking and pill popping aside, the 1930s offered dieters a range of possibilities. Alongside inevitable variations on the low-carb, high-protein theme was a new and novel alternative: the Hay Diet.

Also known as 'food combining', the Hay Diet was introduced by New York physician and nutritionist Dr William Howard Hay in 1911, but it took until the mid-1930s for Dr Hay to become a household name. Despite this slow acceptance, the diet has stood the test of time and many people – including, reportedly, celebrities such as Catherine Zeta Jones and Elizabeth Hurley – still follow Hay's principles today.

Dr Hay contended that *how* you ate was as important as *what* you ate. He said that, because starches and proteins are digested differently, eating them together slowed down digestion, making weight loss more difficult, while all that undigested food lingering in the body would lead to a build-up of toxins and, eventually, disease.

The solution was never to eat proteins and starches within four hours of each other 'for instance, if you are eating starches, you don't eat proteins at the same meal; if it is fruit you are consuming, you skip the starches', Grace Wilcox of *The Milwaukee Journal* explained to her readers in 1935. Instead of eating meat and potatoes together, Hay dieters should combine each group only with 'neutral' foods like vegetables, nuts and seeds.

> '**Today many of the stars are following the Hay Diet,
> which was originated at the Hay sanatorium.**'
>
> – *Grace Wilcox, Milwaukee Journal, November 24, 1935*

Like many modern diets – and in sharp contrast to most of the available alternatives – the Hay Diet was not a quick-fix fad but rather a lifestyle change. The diet could certainly result in weight loss in cases where there were extra pounds to be shed – Hay himself lost considerable poundage adhering to his own plan, and kept it off – but the aim of the plan was to improve overall health rather than to reduce proportions. In the health-conscious 1930s, Dr Hay's diet was *the* programme to follow – with Hollywood leading the way.

RULES OF THE HAY DIET

1. Eat sparingly and only when hungry.
2. Only eat foods that are nourishing.
3. Avoiding pairing foods that cannot easily be digested together (i.e. protein and carbohydrates).
4. Choose foods high in alkali (e.g. lemons, olive oil or asparagus) over acidic foods (e.g. white flour, cheese or beef).

Vintage Expert's Opinion: 'These diets, of course, are relatively harmless, except that it is a nuisance to eat them. The worst difficulty is that the person who is sick will try to cure himself by using one of these diets, without finding out what is really wrong.' – Dr Morris Fishbein, M.D., Editor, *Journal of the American Medical Association*.

Modern Expert's Opinion: 'Our results substantiate the lack of benefit of dissociated [food combining] vs. balanced diets in terms of weight loss and further support that it is energy intake [i.e. how many calories you take in] not energy composition [i.e. how the food is combined] . . . that determines weight loss in response to low-energy diets.' – *International Journal of Obesity*, 2000

THE BANANAS AND
SKIMMED MILK DIET

*'When a star has to take a camera test these days,
she goes on bananas and skimmed milk for one week
and comes out seven pounds thinner to a dot.'*
– *Mollie Merrick, North American Newspaper Alliance, May 9, 1934*

In the 1930s, the banana overtook the grapefruit as the diet food of choice in Hollywood – and everywhere else. The milk cure had been around since the turn of the century, but when Dr George Harrop decided to throw bananas into the mix he created a new sensation. Originally created as a treatment for diabetes at John Hopkins University, the diet soon spread across the US – and the world – as the fad diet of the moment. Dr Harrop gave the dieter the option of two different banana and milk-based plans: one for gradual weight loss, the other providing a more rapid reduction.

The first diet was a moderate 1000-1200 calorie regimen designed for slow and steady reducing. This diet could be employed indefinitely by 'adults whose overweight has been due to overeating', wrote Lois Leeds of the *Boston Globe*. The menu involved a breakfast and lunch of (you guessed it) bananas and skimmed milk and a dinner of clear consommé, a small portion of watery vegetables, and lean meat (fish or fowl), followed by bread with butter and uncooked fruit.

The second option was a three-phase diet in the manner of many modern weight-loss plans such as the Atkins or Dukan diets. Each phase lasted a period of ten days to two weeks.

In the first phase, the dieter was allowed just 940 calories per day, resulting in a predicted weight loss of four to nine pounds in 'persons who lead a moderately active life'. The daily menu allowed only six large, ripe bananas and four half-pint glasses of skimmed milk (or buttermilk) as well as six large glasses of 'liquid without food value', which might include water or tea or coffee without cream or sugar. During this period, the diet's creator does allow some mineral oil to combat the seemingly inevitable constipation. Monsieur Dukan might call this phase 'attack'.

The second phase of the plan is slightly less restrictive. Having become sick of the sight of bananas, the dieter is now permitted to substitute one or two of these for one or two eggs (steamed or poached) and a one-quarter square of butter. One to four servings of 'succulent green vegetables' are also permitted, with a whole square of butter (added *after* cooking). A small portion of lean meat, fish or poultry (plain and unseasoned; never pork) rounds off the day.

The final phase sees the return of bananas and milk for breakfast, lunch and dinner once again. If necessary or desired, the dieter may then repeat this alternating system on and off until the required weight loss has been achieved or, as *The Milwaukee Journal* put it in 1934, until 'you break down and cry at the sight of a banana'.

'Yes, yes, our good plump friends, you may try the banana diet safely for the purpose of reducing and you may be fairly sure of results.'

– Claud North Chrisman, M.D., Berkeley Daily Gazette, May 29, 1935

As always, many doctors had their doubts about this fad diet, but it retained popularity. Dietician and health columnist Ida Jean Kain first alerted her readers to the Banana and Milk plan in 1936 and was still heartily endorsing the diet in the late 1940s. Like so many fad diets, this one also resurfaced in the 1980s.

Vintage Expert's Opinion: 'That the banana is a filling food is a matter of common knowledge. Milk, in itself almost a complete food, makes in combination with the banana a simple, palatable, nutritious and balanced diet.' – Dr Iago Galdston, *Spokane Daily Chronicle*, 1934

Modern Expert's Opinion: 'Anyone following this calorie-restricted plan would undoubtedly lose weight – and gain it back again as soon as he or she went back to a normal diet.' – Susan Yager (Adjunct Professor of Nutrition, Food Studies and Public Health at New York University), *The Hundred Year Diet*

Jean Harlow's

FOUR-DAY DIET

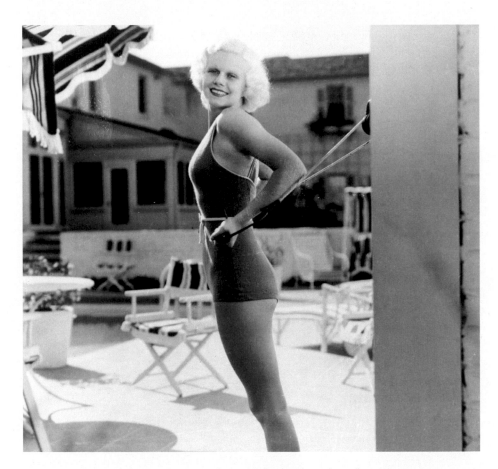

'It is much easier to keep a daily check on one's
measurements and weight and to rectify any creeping-
up inches or pounds than to ignore one's body
until the added flesh takes possession.'

– Jean Harlow

The original Platinum Blonde, Jean Harlow inspired a generation of women, including a certain Norma Jeane Mortenson (later to become famous as Marilyn Monroe), to bleach their hair and don sexy bias-cut dresses that emphasised their curves. Jean was just 5'2" and, at her screen-ready best, she weighed 109 pounds, distributed over a curvy 33-25-35 figure. She was naturally sporty, but she struggled to keep that made-for-satin figure in check.

Jean was a yo-yo dieter. While filming she would stick to vegetables and cottage cheese but between movies she preferred beef stew or chicken à la king. Inevitably, she would be required to drop a few pounds before each new movie, and she relied on this special four-day diet – a sort of early Atkins regime of her own devising – to 'fix' her figure. Jean's tomato-based meal plan soon gained popularity throughout Hollywood with others who needed to shed weight fast. The idea was that you would lose around six pounds if you stuck to the diet for four days and more if you could hack it for longer. Revealingly, Jean cautions that you really shouldn't employ this diet more than once a month.

Breakfast: Black coffee <u>then</u> orange juice.

Lunch (first three days): Two broiled lamb chops; two whole tomatoes (with salt and pepper). Black coffee. Half a grapefruit (after eating).

Dinner Day 1: One grilled sirloin steak, two tomatoes. Black coffee. Orange juice (after eating).

Dinner Day 2: One grilled lamb chop; one dish spinach; one hard boiled egg; two tomatoes. Black coffee. Orange juice (after eating).

Dinner Day 3: Scrambled eggs; two tomatoes. Fruit jello. Black coffee. Orange juice.

Lunch Day 4: Half a fried chicken; two tomatoes. Black coffee. Orange juice.

Dinner Day 4: Two lamb chops; two tomatoes. Black coffee. Orange juice.

Marlene Dietrich

THE DIETRICH DIET

'Health Food: It doesn't sound good;
it tastes good, feels good and does good.'

– Marlene Dietrich

Beautiful, elegant and aloof, it's hard to imagine Marlene Dietrich as anything other than the enigmatic goddess of the screen. Hollywood, of course, found her too healthy and hearty when she first arrived in town. She was encouraged to lose weight and she did so – a diet of tomato juice and crackers apparently did the trick – but she returned to her usual German favourites once the pounds had been shed. And she never put them back on. Marlene found exercise 'boring', but like many who lived through the privations of the First World War, she understood the importance of a good meal. She frequented fashionable health food stores but cooked simple, nutritious meals for herself and her family. She was a huge fan of practical sandwiches – made with good German rye bread, naturally.

MARLENE'S SHOPPING LIST

Artichoke: 'Great remedy for the overworked liver . . . Just try eating a couple of artichokes instead of lunch and dinner and watch your headache disappear.'

Liverwurst: 'It will chase the stomach's butterflies away and also give a good push to the black clouds that make life seem too dark to bear.'

Apples: 'Sad people don't eat apples and people who don't feel well don't eat apples.'

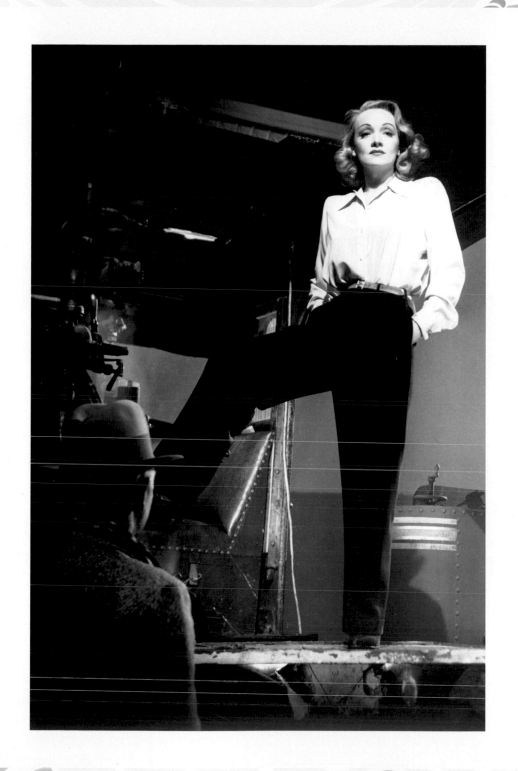

HOLLYWOOD'S BODY SCULPTORS

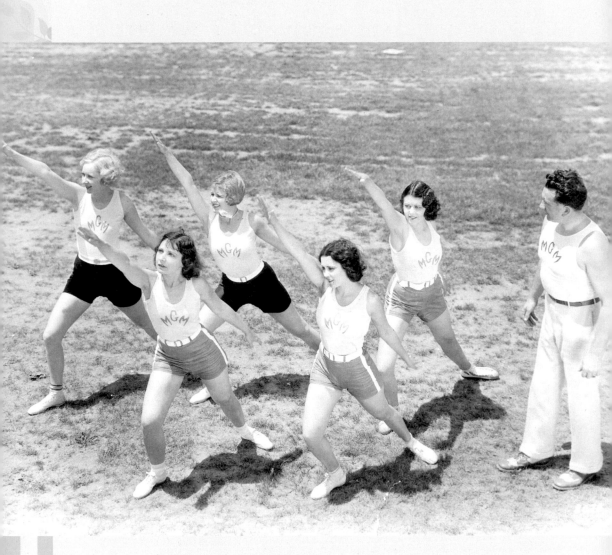

'Proper exercise makes diets unnecessary.'
– Donald Loomis

In the golden age of Hollywood, stars' bodies were their paycheques and a few extra pounds could cost an actress her contract. Many studios built gyms on the lot and hired physical directors to help the stars shape up. These 'muscle men' worked with an array of actors and actresses: some younger, some older; some inclined to put on weight and others in need of a few more pounds. Each star had his or her own goals and each fitness guru had his own methods. From the more traditional routines – calisthenics and rope skipping – favoured by the likes of Donald Loomis at MGM, to the more theatrical methods – Indian war dances and donkey kicks – employed by Paramount's Richard Kline. Naturally, the workout had to be tailored to the star: while Jean Harlow must work 'to diminish her hips', singer Jeanette MacDonald lifted bar weights to increase her diaphragm. Whatever the problem, you could be sure the studio's resident 'flesh sculptor' would find a solution.

DON LOOMIS'S GOLDEN FITNESS RULES

Star clients included: Jean Harlow, Joan Crawford, Katharine Hepburn, and Ginger Rogers.

'Health Trainer Don Loomis is physical father confessor to the most glamorous stars in Hollywood.' – The Milwaukee Journal, 1936

1: Don't diet and especially avoid 'freak diets'.

2: Start the day with a glass of warm water with the juice of one lemon.

3: Take deep breathing exercises before an open window, followed by a tepid shower – not too warm nor too cold.

4: Don't add salt: 'Most foods contain sufficient natural salts.'

5: Be sure to get eight hours sleep.

6: Weight lost too quickly will come back quickly: 'The secret is to build up muscle to take its place.'

'Symmetry is the objective of Hollywood body sculptors.'

– Literary Digest, March 6, 1937

DICK KLINE'S 'FUN' EXERCISES

Star clients included: Betty Grable, Claudette Colbert, Carole Lombard, and Dorothy Lamour.

'In Dick Kline's gymnasium we find the round-faced lassie doing the bird-pecking exercise to take away that pudgy look, slenderise her neck and help her keep its youthful lines.' – The Picturegoer Summer Annual, *1938*

To slenderise the neck and reduce a double chin:

Bird-Pecking: Purse the mouth and peck forward with chin and mouth 'like an eager young bird'. Making bird noises at the same time makes this exercise more fun!

'I will! I won't!': Tilt head back and then drop the head with a little snap as you declare, 'I will!' Turn the head slightly to the right and snap it to the left as you cry, emphatically, 'I won't!'

For a slender waist and beautiful arms:

The Bargain Basement: (Whilst shouting 'Out of my way! I want that bargain!') twist at the waist, pushing away obstructions (and other customers) with bent arms.

The Shakespeare: Stalk about the 'stage', gesticulating in old-fashioned, melodramatic style. Fling those arms to the rafters!

They Torture THEMSELVES to be beautiful

Glamour Girls of the Screen go through all sorts of hard physical stunts to acquire "The Perfect Figure" much they must have. Nevertheless you'll find this article on how they achieve that perfection helpful in your own problems as well as an absorbingly interesting glimpse behind the scenes.

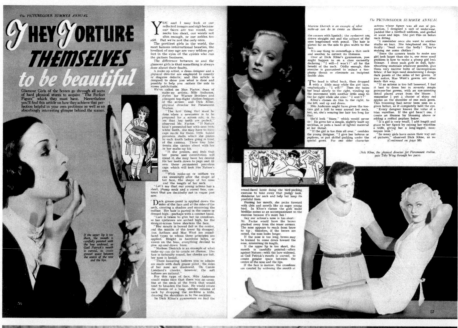

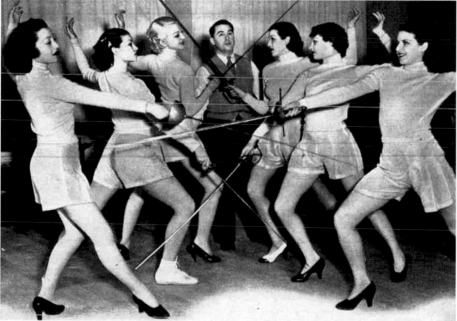

Hollywood's physical directors divulge fitness tricks of the trade. **Above:** Dick Kline of Paramount runs a private fitness session for a young starlet. **Below:** Kline's studio rival, Dance Director Le Roy Prinz, puts his 'children' through their paces.

Ginger Rogers

DANCING FOR HER LIFE

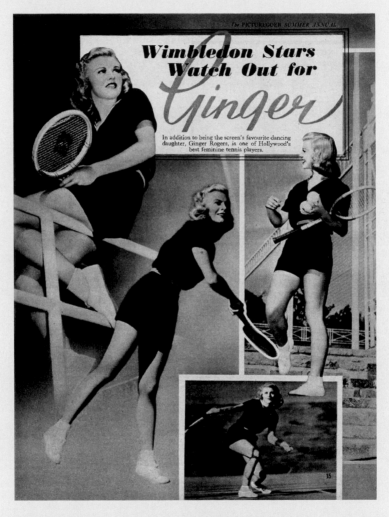

'Ginger is one of Hollywood's most perfect
examples of what exercise will do for a girl.'
– *Ida Jean Kain, Beauty Columnist*

'If you asked Ginger Rogers how to keep healthy, how to keep young, how to have a perfect figure, how to hold a husband or how to be happy, the honest answer would be exactly the same to all questions: Dance.'

– Adela Rogers St Johns, Physical Culture Magazine, 1937

Ginger Rogers had perhaps the perfect 1930s figure: 'She is not thin,' *The Milwaukee Sentinel* pointed out in 1941. 'She is slim and her weight is beautifully distributed.' Hers was a figure built on plenty of good food and physical exercise. During the filming – and practicing – of complicated dance routines, Ginger worked so hard that even her hearty, southern-girl diet of chicken and 'cowboy' gravy didn't stop her losing weight. Off-screen, Ginger was always on the go: she got a kick out of tennis, and was crazy about badminton and ping-pong. She'd try anything once. Golf is the only sport Ginger doesn't seem to have taken to with enthusiasm. 'Just as well,' she shrugged. 'I probably wouldn't have any time to make movies!'

Of course, Ginger's favourite form of exercise was dancing, to which she attributed not only her lovely figure but also all the health and happiness she enjoyed in life: 'If you take the same hour to dance that you take for routine exercise, what have you got? First of all, you learn how to dance and dance well, and that's a great joy in itself. Second, you develop grace while you are developing muscular control and that's important to a woman because grace is the first essential of charm. Then, because you dance to music, your mind and body coordinate and cooperate and so your whole being gets the benefit.'

And, according to Ginger, you can have all that too. Talent isn't important in her book. Like today's Zumba craze, which promises 'a total-body workout that feels like a celebration', Ginger swears the dancing is the key, not whether you get the steps right or wrong. Her advice for ordinary women of ordinary talent is: 'Do whatever you want to do . . . I'd go somewhere and dance as often as I could but I'd dance by myself in my own room every single day and I'd just have a glorious time doing it.'

Ginger's Top Tip: Don't cross your legs! According to Ginger, crossing one's legs 'will change the muscles and make you look like you're riding a horse the whole time.'

LUNCHTIME IN HOLLYWOOD

'The reason foreign actresses seldom enjoy lasting careers in Hollywood can be traced to their taste for rich food and plenty of it . . . Many European imports have literally eaten their way off the screen.'

– The Hartford Courant, 1941

During a busy working day, the responsibility of keeping the studio's most precious assets in top condition resided with the managers of the studio commissaries. The likes of MGM's Frances Edwards or Katherine Higgins, who presided over Warner Bros' Green Room, became amateur dieticians, catering carefully to the wants, needs, and whims of the stars in their care.

The Café de Paris at 20th Century Fox – generally considered the best of the studio restaurants – was ruled over by flamboyant Nick Janios for over 30 years. Nick took his responsibilities very seriously, weighing out every portion on special scales, counting the calories, obeying stars' individual diet lists down to the last drop of mineral oil.

According to the commissary staff, most of the younger actresses rarely dieted – apparently tomatoes and cottage cheese is classed as a 'light lunch' – and burnt off excess fat through hard work and nervous energy. At the very least, most of these glamorous young ladies were seen to

'Gals sit in restaurants with heaping plates of food before them, in place of the green salad and glass of buttermilk of other days. But watch closely my friends. They nibble spinach off the corner of the plate and make a lot of gestures with the rest of that gargantuan luncheon.'

– Molly Merrick, North American Newspaper Alliance, 1934

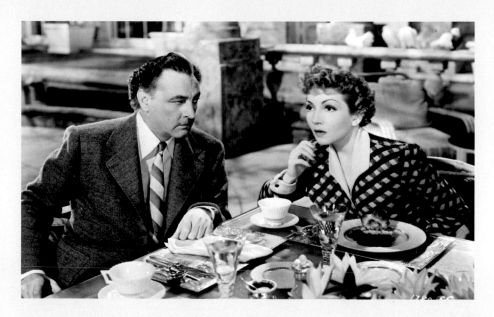

'Most of our stars find that light lunches
keep them more alert during production.'

– Hazel Moore, Paramount Restaurant Manager

take plenty of food – even if they didn't necessarily tuck in. But for those who had passed 30 – and were still lucky enough to be sought after in 'glamour' roles – lunchtime was not so carefree. These 'ageing' beauties had to watch their calories – and those extra potatoes – or risk losing their leading-lady status altogether. The message to fan-magazine readers was that to be young was to be beautiful: ageing and gaining weight (at this time, virtually synonymous terms) were to be avoided at all costs.

Perhaps because they had not yet learned the American art of disdaining diet whilst abstaining from food, foreign stars had a reputation for large appetites, extravagant tastes and a tendency to put on weight. Even the glorious Hedy Lamarr, in her willowy prime, was said to resort to diets after the 'European' tendency to overeat got the better of her. It was this foreign failing, Harold Heffernan of *The Hartford Courant* suggests, that resulted in the short shelf-lives of many imported Hollywood stars. Though the 1930s woman was encouraged to avoid extreme thinness and fad diets, she was also constantly reminded that beauty and success (in Hollywood and elsewhere) depended on a slender body.

INSIDE

Bette Davis's

LUNCH BOX

O ver on the Warner Bros lot, Joan Crawford's arch-nemesis Bette Davis was making sacrifices to keep slim. Nicknamed 'spuds' at school for her love of mashed potato, the divine Miss Davis resolutely turned down these and many of her other favourite foods in order to maintain her fantastic figure (and rival queen bee status). Alert to the dangers of a busy schedule, she always had a *healthy* snack on hand in case her stomach started rumbling before lunchtime.

Bette had friends in the right places: the studio café to be precise. Manager Katherine Higgins and her staff loved the easy-going star and always made sure she had what she wanted for lunch, prepared just the way she liked it. She would order a variety of foods but, like so many girls in Hollywood, she never finished any of the dishes.

Bette, who once had a job as a lifeguard, also believed that swimming every day helped her maintain good overall fitness. In particular, she attributed her lovely legs and slim waist to the scissor leg movement. Dancing and riding were also part of her active lifestyle.

BETTE'S SLIMMING SNACKS

Hearts of celery with salt (celery kills cravings; salt adds taste).

Raisins (for a healthy sugar hit).

Romaine leaves in oil dressing (light but filling).

A glass of water every hour (healthy, filling, and calorie free!).

Working Lunch (at the Warner Bros Café): Endive salad, calves liver and bacon, fruit salad, milk. Cigarettes.

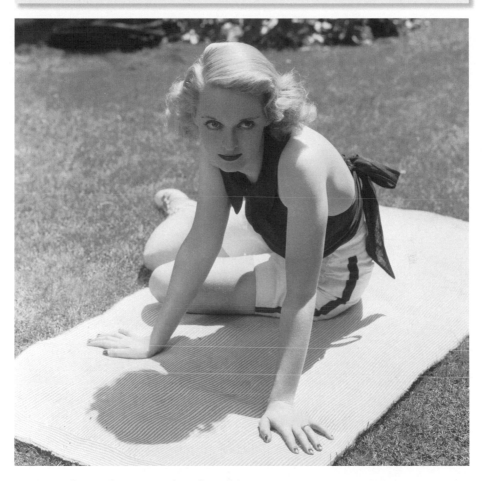

'Today, the new look of beauty is an inspiring one.
There may be prettiness to it, but never vacuously
pretty. It's the look of radiant health stemming from
physical and mental wellbeing and, above all,
a look of being capable as well as feminine.'

– *Bette Davis*

1940s
Pin-Up Proportions

'If any considerable number of women are
questioned directly as to why they have reduced their
weights, it is not likely that many of them will reply
honestly that they reduced to improve their health.'
– *Dr Morris Fishbein, The Spokane Daily Chronicle, January 2, 1940*

With the world in the grip of another world war, women of
the 1940s had to be simultaneously strong and feminine:
the competent working girl and the sweetheart waiting back
home; mothers of the nation and home-front fighters. At a time when
everybody needed to be fit and healthy and 'do their bit', nutrition
became the watchword for the decade. Calisthenics – requiring no
special equipment or particular skill – enjoyed a popularity boom as
builders of strength and stamina. Girls were still dieting, but they did so
ostensibly to improve their health – of course, it was also their patriotic
duty to look their best for the boys on the frontlines.

The same could be said for Hollywood's leading ladies, suddenly
the sole box-office draw, alongside almost unknown actors, as many
matinee idols went off to fight in Europe. Throughout the war, studios
received thousands of letters from servicemen requesting pin-up shots
of the likes of Betty Grable, Rita Hayworth and Dorothy Lamour. They
wanted to see healthy figures – an idealised likeness of the girl back home
– not distant, super-slim goddesses. Hollywood's glamour girls obliged
by eating up and filling out to suit new, more feminine fashions. Nick

> **'After several years of dieting to produce the fashionable "streamlined" figures, the screen's ladies have decided to look rounder and better fed.'**
>
> *– The Pittsburgh Post Gazette, August 31, 1938*

Janios, still in the kitchens at 20th Century Fox, reported desserts had never been so popular; the costume department confirmed that curves were definitely back.

Everyone, everywhere was working more, walking more, and eating less. With the fashion for curves tempting girls to put on a few pounds and rationing making gaining too much weight less of a danger, there seemed to be very little call for the average girl to actively reduce. The proof that she was still doing so is borne out by a speech from the British Minister for Food, Lord Woolton, in 1942, imploring women to eat more potatoes and assuring them that they simply couldn't get fat on the meagre luxuries allowed by their ration books. But of course the ideal figure, like those of the Hollywood beauties, required not just a beautiful bust but a tiny waist too. It would not be long before the hourglass figure was back in fashion.

The publication of MetLife's charts for ideal heights and weights in 1943 underlined the link between a good figure and good health – and gave women something else to measure up against besides their friends and Hollywood movie queens. Bodily perfection became statistically measurable. Naturally, girls wanted to conform to the standard. What was more, the arrival of ready-to-wear clothing around this time brought with it added pressures to fit into 'fashionable' sizes. Many of the fashions, of course, were set in Hollywood and ready-to-wear meant girls could copy their favourite stars even more closely.

The 1940s delivered more freedom and opportunity for women. But the war years also brought with them an increased pressure to conform to a recognised standard of beauty. Whether dieting towards a healthy BMI or attempting to squeeze ourselves into a skinny size zero, our need to conform to the 'right' size and weight is a legacy of the 1940s.

1940s

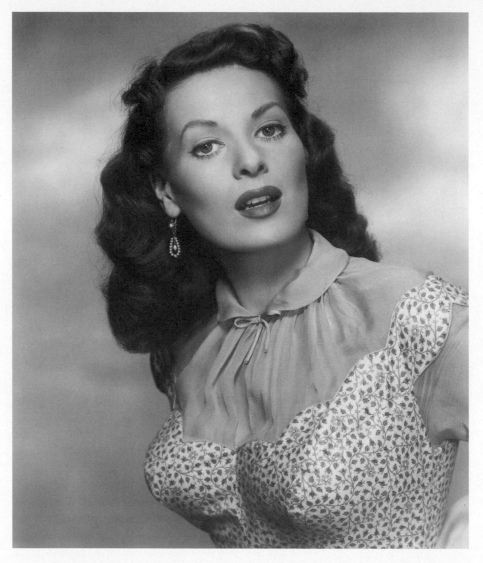

'For years we've worn boyish these and mannish those, which made it necessary to keep thin. . . Now we've gone back to feminine clothes and can look like girls again. I'm all for it. Besides, it means I can have my chocolate sundae with my lunch.'
– *Maureen O'Hara*

CALISTHENICS FOR EVERYONE

Calisthenics enjoyed huge popularity in the forties and were practiced everywhere from Italy to the USA, from army quads to school gyms. They're back in fashion again today, especially with business travellers: you don't need any equipment; you don't need much time or space; they're a cardiovascular workout; and they tone and strengthen. Greta Garbo did them – and so can you.

THE OFFICE GIRL'S EXERCISE PROGRAMME

As men went off to war, 1940s women were increasingly asked to fill their shoes. 'They will have to work just as efficiently and for just as many hours as the men did,' warned beauty columnist Ida Jean Kain in 1942. To help these working gals out, Ida shared 'the office girl's exercise programme', to rouse the circulation, prevent stooping, and combat the 'desk chair spread'.

1. Stand, feet apart and arms at sides. Raise yourself up on your toes and fling your arms out and up at the sides. Swing arms back, letting them cross in front, as you lower your heels to the floor. Repeat twenty times.

2. Stand as before. Pull up with the stomach muscles and stretch through the midriff. Fling arms up and out at sides and swing your left leg straight out at the side. Keep knees straight, swing from the hip. Repeat ten times.

3. Stretch arms overhead and clasp hands, palms turned outward, feet apart. Hold the upstretch through the middle and bend directly sideward. Stretch straight again, and bend to the other side.

4. Swing down to one side and touch hands to the floor outside your foot. Stretch again, and swing down to the other side.

Adapted from: 'Tips for the Girl Who Works', Ida Jean Kain, *The Milwaukee Sentinel*, Nov 4, 1942

THE HOMEMAKER'S EXERCISE PROGRAMME

'If housework were only streamlining! But, alack-a-day it's just plain work . . . You homemakers need calisthenics just as much as the office girls.'

– Ida Jean Kain, nutritionist, 1942

1940s housewives were active all day, burning, today's studies show, up to 1000 calories a day during their daily chores. But even these busy ladies could not escape the forties fervour for calisthenics.

Unfortunately, Ida explained, homemakers were using only *small* muscles as they dusted, swept and ironed – that's bad news for the waist and hips, ladies. There was some reprieve, however: because they were on their feet all day, Ida let housewives lie down to exercise.

According to Ida, this fifteen-minute routine 'will put you in such good shape that you can romp through your housework and have energy leftover to do your share in defence [of the nation]'.

1. Lie on back, knees bent and feet on floor. Pull stomach muscles up and in and press small of back flat against the floor. Hold for a second and relax. Repeat ten times.

2. In the same position, flex alternate knees to chest. Repeat ten times.

3. Elevate your feet to the seat of a low chair, legs straight. From that position, repeat exercise.

4. Finish with the side-scissors. Lie on your side in a straight line. Swing the legs from the hips in a scissors action. Continue for 50 counts. Variation: keeping the under leg still, swing the top leg out in front and up and out in back.

Adapted from: 'Exercise for Home Makers' by Ida Jean Kain, *The Milwaukee Sentinel*, Nov 3, 1942

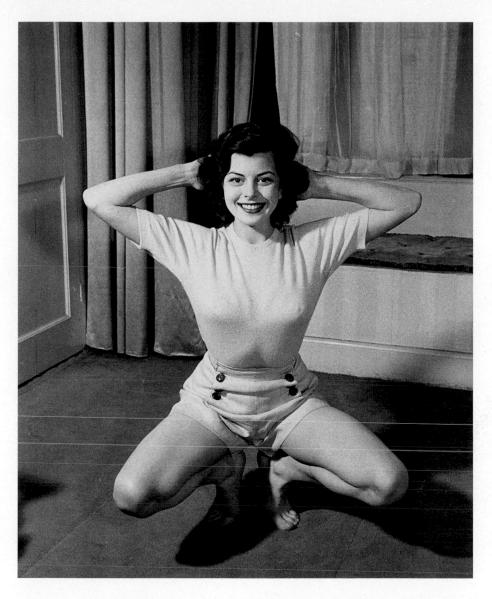

'Don't skip exercise entirely and think you can go on working at
top speed. It will gradually cut down on your efficiency.
Your brain and nerves get tired, but you need a healthy physical
fatigue. The only way you can get it is through a set of exercises.'

– *Ida Jean Kain, nutritionist, 1942*

Betty Grable

TAKING CARE OF
MILLION-DOLLAR LEGS

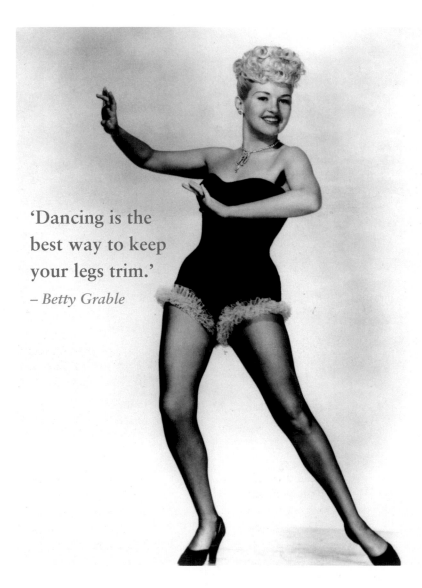

'Dancing is the
best way to keep
your legs trim.'
– *Betty Grable*

> *'The boys like her for her lines*
> *and she doesn't have to read them.'*
>
> *– Photoplay, June 1943*

The most popular pin-up of the Second World War, Betty Grable famously declared, 'There are two reasons why I'm in show business – and I'm standing on both of them.' Jokes aside, the girl with the million-dollar legs certainly owed a lot to her perfect pins. So famous that they were immortalised in concrete at Grauman's Chinese Theatre, Betty's beautiful limbs also ensured her plenty of screen time. With fabric subject to rationing, it cost the studio less to make her outfits, while the sight of her best assets boosted the troops' morale! Betty was smart enough to take good care of her money-winners.

Betty also took good care of her overall health: her favourite snacks were onions and garlic, which she rightly believed were pretty good for her. She also believed in beauty sleep and insisted on getting eight hours, regardless of when she came in from dancing the night away. She must have been doing something right because, in spite of garlic-breath, there was no star more sought after in the 1940s.

BETTY'S TIPS FOR BEAUTIFUL LEGS

Tip #1: Dance! According to Betty, 'Dancing is the best way to keep your legs trim.' She recommended starting young: 'Because I started early, I never went through the awkward stage.'

Tip #2: Walk! 'Legs, you know, were meant for walking and since gas rationing many of us are luckily learning to use them more often.'

Tip #3: Get the blood flowing! Betty recommended massage every night to improve your circulation: 'Start at the toes and work the tiredness out with a rotary motion. Then with both palms flat against ankles, massage gently at least 40 times. Above the ankle, use a brisk up and down movement that will circulate the blood.'

Ann Sheridan's

TIPS FOR GIRLS WHO DARE TO BARE

'Ann Sheridan believes some thought
ought to be given to the beauty of the midriff
since the boundaries of complexion
have been definitely extended.'

– The Reading Eagle, 1940

While governments urged people to 'Make, do, and mend', Hollywood responded to textile rationing by wearing less. From cropped (v-neck, sleeveless) sweaters, to bare-midriff evening gowns, with more flesh on show, leading ladies had to be sure their bodies were as beautiful as their faces. For Ann Sheridan – whose fabulous figure earned her the nickname 'the oomph girl' – the new European fashion for baring one's belly was not an intimidating prospect. Ann took good care of her body, eating well and exercising regularly. She played tennis and badminton and skated every morning (in stylish, custom-made outfits, of course). Besides a tiny waist, according to photographer George Hurrell, Ann also had 'photographically perfect' shoulders.

FOR PERFECT SHOULDERS

1. Raise arms to shoulder height, making a T shape with the body. Bend arms from the elbow until finger tips touch. Press fingers together, relax, and press together again.

2. Swing both arms in a complete circle clockwise, then anticlockwise.

FOR MIDRIFF-BARERS

1: Morning Exercise. Lie face down; elbows bent, hands – palms down – between chest and bed; legs straight. Keeping legs straight raise yourself upward until elbows are straight and weight is on hands and toes.

2: Embellish. Ann wore body tints to ensure her belly looked its best.

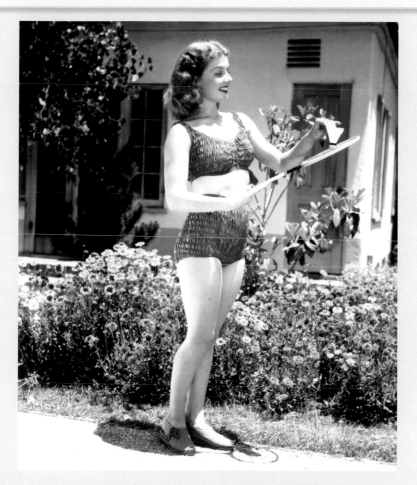

'Exercise is the most important body tuner.'

– Ann Sheridan

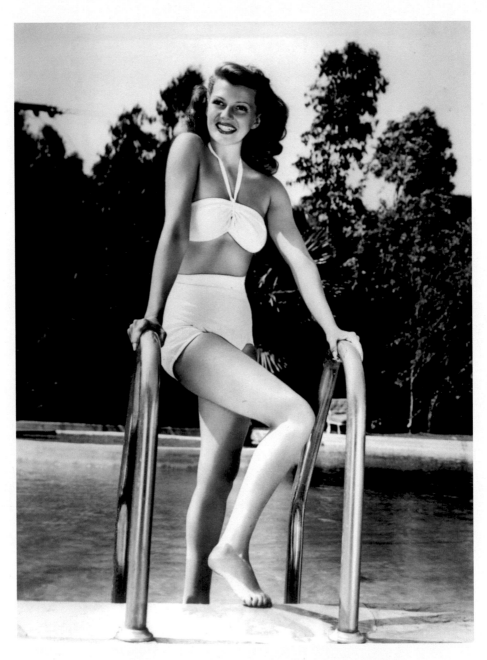

'I believe in reducing the natural way.'
– *Rita Hayworth*

Rita Hayworth

GODDESS GUIDE

> 'Honey, they had me dancing as soon as
> they could get me on my feet.'
>
> – *Rita Hayworth*

Hailed as a goddess, Rita Hayworth was the biggest pin-up of the forties. Once a Hispanic, black-haired beauty by the name of Margarita Carmen Cansino, she would become Hollywood's all-American redhead, the dream girl next door. She was 'The Best Dressed Girl in Hollywood', 'Hollywood's Most Fascinating Woman Number One', the face for dozens of famous brands, selling everything from cosmetics to margarine. By the time she married Prince Aly Khan in 1949, she was so famous that replicas of her wedding dress were available to buy in Macy's. Every girl wanted to look like Rita – so how did she do it?

When asked her reducing secret by 'Hollywood Beauty' columnist Lydia Lane, Rita replied, simply, 'Dancing: eight hours a day.' The response is hardly surprising. Rita came from a family of dancers and started training to enter the family profession at the age of four, learning Spanish dancing, ballet and 'all other kinds of dancing' – and acquiring a graceful, elegant figure along the way.

> 'I eat fairly sensibly. No starches and greasy foods, no heavy bread and pastries.'
>
> – *Rita Hayworth*

Most of her early roles involved musical dance routines, meaning that she kept up her training even when she became a Hollywood star. All this dancing meant that Rita never really needed to diet. When Rita and Fred Astaire were preparing for *You'll Never Get Rich* in 1941, Rita lost 20 lbs. Any weight she put on between films, however, she worked off through the simple strengthening exercises of the Bagot Stack System.

THE BAGOT STACK STRETCH AND SWING SYSTEM

Long before aerobics and step, there was Bagot Stack. Mary Bagot Stack's eponymous fitness method originated in Britain in the 1930s as an exercise programme for the average woman: inexpensive, requiring no special equipment, and providing a complete body workout. Her classes combined dance with exercise, putting emphasis on the rhythm of movement.

By the start of the Second World War, the popular 'stretch and swing' classes had spread to Canada and Australia – and acquired 200,000 followers along the way. In 1941, Rita introduced American girls to the routines she herself practiced. She recommended learning all the moves, then creating your own repertoire, tailored to your body.

The Bagot Stack method is still taught worldwide today. But anyone attending an inexpensive group exercise class should thank Molly Bagot Stack.

ANKLE SPRINGING (FOR THIGHS AND LEGS)

Position: Stand holding the back of a straight chair.

Exercise: Spring from ankles up onto toes, raising heels high. Return to starting position, spring up again. *Do not use your arms; make the ankles do the work*. Repeat until you can get way up on the tips of your toes – as a ballet dancer does.

Part Two: Repeat exercise without the chair, and without losing balance. Stand, feet flat on floor, head up. Fix eyes on an object at eye-level. Spring! Push from the heels up onto tiptoes but come quickly down again. Practice for ten minutes at least.

Adapted from 'Calling All Women!', Hope Chandler, *The Daily Boston Globe*, Mar 24, 1941.

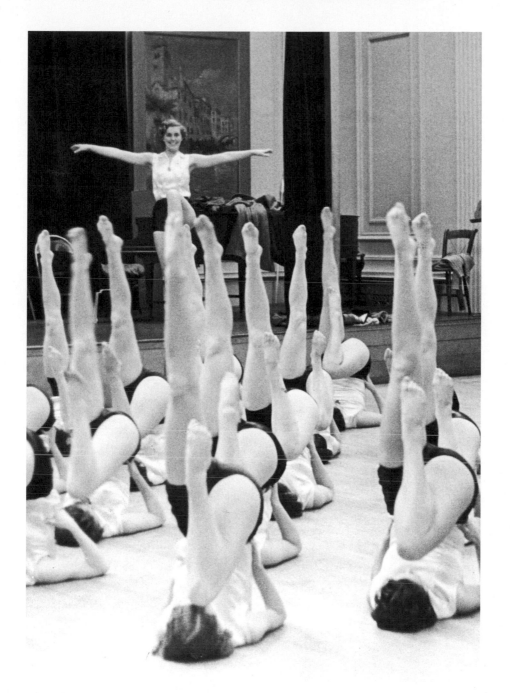

Above: In full swing: A group of British girls practice the Bagot-Stack fitness method in the late 1930s.

MEASURING DESIRE
THE (STATISTICALLY) IDEAL FIGURE

When Met Life introduced 'desirable' height and weight tables in 1943, they inevitably sparked a debate on the subject of 'ideal' figures. Although the insurance company's reports, based on millions of policies, aimed to pinpoint those likely to live longest, beauty columnists were more interested in aesthetically pleasing proportions.

MET LIFE'S 'DESIRABLE' WOMAN 1943

Height	Small Frame	Medium Frame	Large Frame
5' 0"	105-113	112-120	119-129
5' 1"	107-115	114-122	121-131
5' 2"	110-118	117-125	124-135
5' 3"	113-121	120-128	127-138
5' 4"	116-125	124-132	131-142
5' 5"	119-128	127-135	133-145
5' 6"	123-132	130-140	138-150
5' 7"	126-136	134-144	142-154
5' 8"	129-139	137-147	145-158
5' 9"	133-143	141-151	149-162
5' 10"	136-147	145-155	152-166
5' 11"	139-150	148-158	155-169
6' 0"	141-153	151-163	160-174

Weights for women over 25 lbs (in clothing weighing 3 lbs; in shoes with 1" heels)

HOW HOLLYWOOD
MEASURED UP

Over in Hollywood, studio physical directors like Jim Davies of Paramount and Louis Hippe at Warner Bros had their own – far more specific – ideas about what made the ideal woman. For one thing, she needed to weigh ten pounds less in real life than she wanted to appear on-screen . . .

While many silver-screen sirens fit comfortably into Met Life's 'desirable' weight range for their height – maybe a few pounds lighter – few of them met the Hollywood exercise gurus' more exacting standards:

Rita Hayworth, while a little too tall and too light at 5'6" and 120 lbs, could have benefitted from losing two inches off her bust and hips.

HOLLYWOOD'S IDEAL FIGURE	
Height	5'5"
Weight	125 lbs
Bust	34"
Waist	24"
Hips	34"
Thigh	21"
Knee	13 ½"
Calf	12 ½"
Ankle	8"

Veronica Lake, just 5'1", was too short for perfect beauty, and her astonishing 34-18.5-34 figure was far too curvy.

Katharine Hepburn, despite her pound-a-week chocolate habit, was too skinny.

Lana Turner, who started every movie ten pounds overweight (before nerves – or something else – knocked off those extra pounds), measured up almost perfectly.

Dorothy Lamour's
PERFECT PROPORTIONS

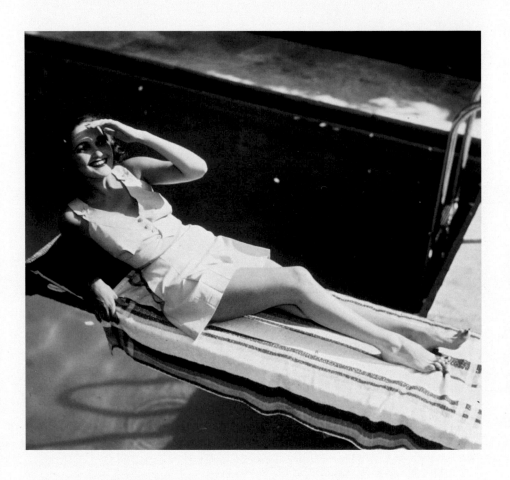

'I think that three exercises – one for hips,
another for waistline and one for the chest muscles
– keep my figure in good shape.'

– Dorothy Lamour

'A "glamour girl" must have a figure to catch the eye.
If diet and exercise are needed to keep it that way,
then, for heaven's sake, do both.'

– Dorothy Lamour

One girl who had the experts – and the boys on the front lines – in perfect agreement was popular pin-up Dorothy Lamour. Everyone agreed that her pounds balanced beautifully over those three, all-important points: hips, waist, and chest. No wonder she looked so good in a sarong. And far from relying on the tricks of the trade, by all accounts Dottie was even lovelier in real life. Despite rumours that she lived off a 'jungle diet' of coconut, bananas and pineapples, for the most part Hollywood's favourite 'native girl' stuck to healthy, balanced meals and avoided fads. To maintain her beautiful figure, she swore by a special exercise programme devised for her by Paramount's health and exercise guru, Jim Davies.

THE PERFECT PIN-UP ROUTINE

Hips: Lie on floor with arms folded. Keeping ankles together, lift feet about four inches from floor; at the same time, lift head and shoulders lightly, shifting weight onto hips. Roll to the right until you face the floor, then once over again, until facing the ceiling. Now two rolls left. Repeat ten times the first day, adding two rolls every day until you reach 50.

Waistline: Reach for the ceiling, then bend forward to touch the floor. Keeping knees stiff, bend to the left, to the right, then backward as far as possible. The last step is the most important, according to Miss Lamour.

Chest: Hold hands at chest level with elbows up, fingers spread apart with fingertips touching. Quickly press fingertips together, noting how the pectoral muscles of the chest expand. Repeat no more than 40 times a minute for two minutes a day.

Gayelord Hauser

CELEBRITY CHEF

'When you peel, pickle, cook to death or throw away the best parts of food, you are nourishing the kitchen sink and starving your family.'

– Gayelord Hauser

The 1940s saw a huge campaign for healthy living, with several international bestsellers being written on the subject. The war had exposed the low fitness levels – and poor eating habits – of many young men in Europe and America. And new medical studies continued to draw links between food choices, obesity, and disease. All in all, it was an auspicious moment to peddle homeopathic remedies and nature's cures – especially when they were being sold with the flash and charm of Gayelord Hauser.

German-born Benjamin Gayelord Hauser (who claimed to be Viennese because it sounded more glamorous) began promoting healthy eating in Hollywood in the late 1920s and later gained publicity as a dietician to the stars, especially Greta Garbo, who became a walking advertisement for his way of living. By 1940, Hauser was *the* diet guru of Hollywood – and an omnipresent, charismatic media personality (with an attractive, broken accent and a permanent wave).

'In Hollywood, people are very vain, and are more interested in reducing than in health. I am not a beautician.'

– Gayelord Hauser

Hauser was an advocate of whole foods, unrefined sugar and flour, and super foods like alfalfa sprouts and wheat germ. Today, many of his views are middle of the road: he believed in eating a vegetable-heavy diet but thought strict vegetarianism was too extreme; he didn't believe in giving up all one's indulgences but thought you should fill up on food

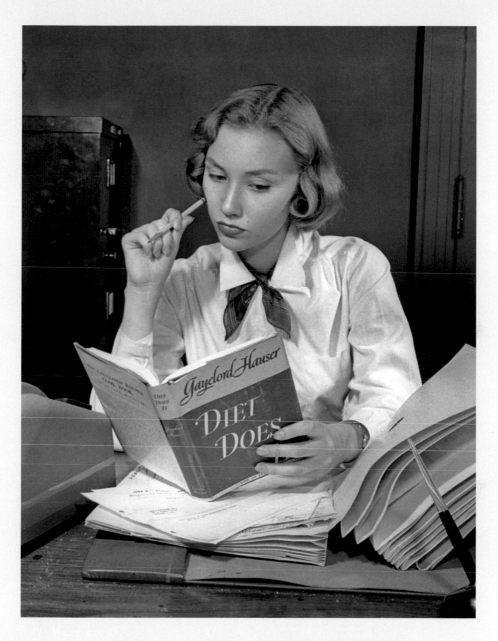

'You must first eat what you need
– then what you want at the dinner table.'

– Gayelord Hauser

> ### 'Man has been asking for trouble since he began tampering with Nature's foodstuffs.'
> *– Gayelord Hauser*

that was good for you before you allowed yourself a treat. Hauser didn't believe in fad diets – he wanted his followers to change their lifestyles forever – but he was a fan of periodic detoxes, like his famous One-Day Beauty Diet, to maintain optimum health.

Gayelord Hauser did not hold a medical degree and his main qualification seems to have been having cured himself of tuberculosis. Despite his success with the stars, and no fewer than eighteen bestselling books, the medical authorities hated the self-styled 'food scientist' and accused him of targeting the gullible and vain. This is not entirely fair. If you can get beyond the patronising, self-congratulatory tone and inexplicable penchant for certain dubious health foods (like blackstrap molasses), many of Hauser's proclamations are actually based on common sense. Sure, have dessert if you must, he says, but fill up on greens first. While some of his more grandiose statements would raise eyebrows today, many still see him as a founding father of the health foods movement.

HAUSER'S ONE-DAY DIET
THE ONE-DAY BEAUTY DIET (SOLID FOOD VERSION)

Breakfast: Sliced orange or half grapefruit. Black coffee or herbal tea.

Lunch: Chopped carrot salad with lemon juice dressing and cottage cheese. Vegetable broth or herbal tea sweetened with honey.

Dinner: Spinach, cooked lightly and seasoned with lemon juice. Fresh fruit salad. One dish of natural, unsweetened yoghurt. Black coffee (small) or herbal tea.

Snacks: Mid-morning and mid-afternoon, any fruit except bananas. If hungry in the evening, have more fresh fruit or 'gentle' herbal teas like camomile (caffeine-free) or peppermint (aids digestion).

HAUSER'S ONE-DAY DIET
THE ONE-DAY BEAUTY DIET (LIQUID VERSION)

Breakfast: One large glass of fresh orange or grapefruit juice. Two cups of hot peppermint or papaya tea sweetened with natural honey or 'if you must' one cup of black coffee.

Lunch: Two cups of vegetable broth. One dish of unsweetened yoghurt, sprinkled with cinnamon, nutmeg or blackstrap molasses.

Dinner: Vegetable broth (all you want). Unsweetened yoghurt with cinnamon, nutmeg or blackstrap molasses. Herbal tea flavoured with natural honey.

Snacks: One large glass of celery, carrot or unsweetened apple juice (or a combination of the three) in the mid-morning and afternoon (or more orange/grapefruit juice if you have no fresh vegetables).

'They talk about spinach cocktails, and carrot cocktails, and cabbage cocktails. All that diet business. Greta's terribly interested in dietetics, and it was this mutual interest that first brought them together. Greta had read all of Gayelord's books on diet before she met him. Which, of course, was a wonderful beginning.'

– *Gordon Barrington, Photoplay, September 1940*

DIETS FOR SKINNY GIRLS WITH
Ava Gardner and Co

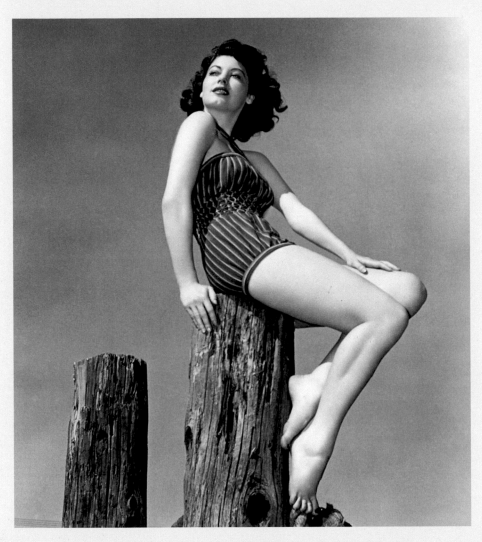

'I have a diet that would put hips on a snake.'
– *Ava Gardner*

'Tension may be contributing to keeping your weight down, no matter how you stuff.'

– Arlene Dahl, Chicago Daily Tribune, Mar 4, 1953

One girl who certainly fit the bill for forties curves was the beautiful and tempestuous Ava Gardner. Ava is as famous for her figure as her wild temper, but maintaining those lovely lines was a constant struggle. Apparently, her 'nervous stomach' made her unable to eat when excited or upset and, as a result, she often lost weight – in spite of an everyday diet of high-calorie foods and portions of pasta that would make most stars blanch.

For many people in the 1940s, Ava's weight struggles seemed natural in one who was famously highly strung. The belief that temperament was a factor in bodyweight was not new and, unlike today's experts, most forties diet pros still believed that the overweight were generally lazy and good natured, while the over-thin were habitually nervous and excitable. Relaxing, then, was a good move for skinny girls. (Unfortunately for nervous smokers, giving up cigarettes was also recommended for those who sought to gain.)

If you simply couldn't relax or, like Ava, your busy schedule never gave you any time to kick back, then a hearty diet of full-fat dairy and assorted carbohydrates was considered a good way to pile on the pounds.

AVA'S CURVE-BUILDING MENU

Breakfast: Bananas and cream; cereal with cream and sugar; 2 rashers of bacon and a fried egg; toast with butter and jam. Coffee or milk.

Lunch: Egg dish; cooked corn; salad with oil or mayonnaise dressing; bread and butter. Bartlett pears with cream. Milk.

Dinner: Creamed soup; steak; creamed potato; fruit salad and dressing. Ice cream and butter cake. Milk.

(Extra) Indulgences: Hershey bars; gum; marshmallows; popcorn; Jack Daniel's; cognac mixed with anise; cigarettes.

1950s
Curves, Curves, Curves

'Monroe's figure is a sign of the times . . .
Women are realising there is nothing wrong
with flesh, particularly when it is in the right places.
It is certainly in the right places on Monroe.'

– Bill Thomas, fashion designer at Universal International

They had proved their mettle during the war, but when husbands and sweethearts began returning home, girls donned their frilliest frocks and most frivolous hats to greet them, making sure their lipstick was perfect, their powder touched up. Returning servicemen wanted to see a *girl*, they were reminded, so show him what you've got! This, in a way, became the spirit of the fifties. Women were returning to traditional roles – for the time being, at least – and fashionable figures reflected this shift. Alluring curves were the order of the day, with Marilyn Monroe and Jane Russell serving as fine examples of the form and only Audrey Hepburn – a forerunner of the 1960s waif – providing an exception to the rule.

Clothes, too, were encouraging an ultra-feminine look. The antithesis of functional wartime garb, fifties fashions emphasised a girl's most womanly assets – bust, waist and hips – and adorned them with girlish frills and bows. Ready-to-wear, now well established in the US and even available for the first time in France, helped to deliver widespread acceptance of the hourglass ideal. 'You too can dress like a star' went the taglines, as advertising and Hollywood ganged up once again to portray the 'perfect'

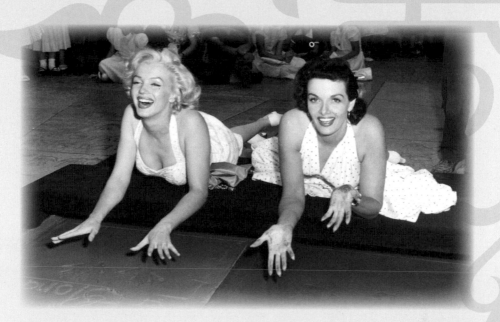

woman. Demanding new styles, as modelled by curvy stars, drew a neat line between the fashionable dress and the ideal form to fill it. Ideally, such ads would run alongside a weight loss regime or exercise plan.

At first glance, the fifties figure, built along more generous lines than in previous decades, should have relieved some of the pressure on women to reduce. Instead, advertising for weight loss aids proliferated and sales of diet books soared throughout the decade as women discovered the difficulties of filling out in just the *right* places. The key to a perfect hourglass figure was achieving 'correct distribution of weight' and this could only

'You can hardly walk a city block these days without

seeing signs of the diet mania, which currently has some

40 million Americans in its grasp.'

– Garven Hudgins,
The St Petersburg Times, 1953

be done (so said the beauty columnists and 'expert' dieticians) through a combination of dieting and 'spot exercises' – today we might call it 'targeting problem areas'.

For those who needed a little help, the corset made a comeback – in the USA, women spent six million dollars on the famous 'Merry Widow' during the 1950s. And, of course, new kinds of diet pills, anti-fat creams and even appetite-suppressant candy all offered hope to those

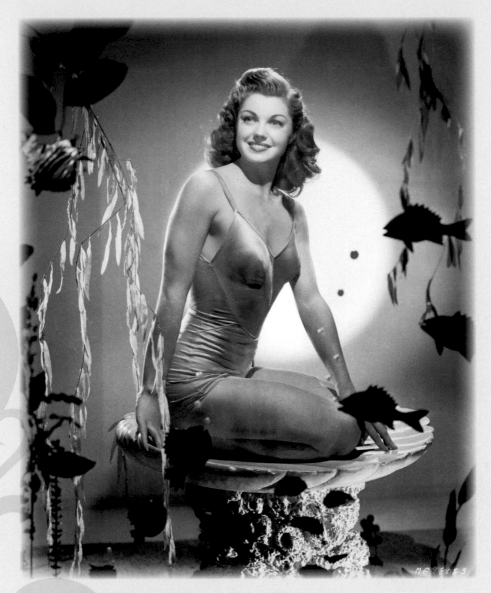

'Whoever heard of a flat-chested mermaid?'

– Esther Williams

who needed to slim down before they shaped up. The fifties even saw
the first TV exercise guru – Jack LaLanne – reaching out to housewives
in their own living rooms, encouraging them to maintain or regain the

'Keep in fashion, do what your friends are doing.
Get on the low-calorie bandwagon.
You may like it – you may even stick to it!'

– St Petersburg Times, July 19, 1953

figure they'd had as a bride. The pressures on women to 'stay young and beautiful' were stronger than ever. This was the first time that weight gain during pregnancy became a widespread concern – as did regaining one's sexuality afterwards. Even stars were happy to talk about how they lost that baby weight.

While during the war most available food had been traditional, basic fare, in the fifties, the rise of convenience foods changed the way people looked at meal times forever. An 'at home' article in *Radioplay* reveals how TV star Joe Mantell, after a very long day at the studio, doesn't come home to a hearty meal being kept hot on the stove. Instead, his blushing young bride lets him raid the icebox for his favourite 'midnight snack'. It's all very modern.

At the same time that convenience foods were becoming more popular – particularly in the USA – diet foods (or 'low-calorie alternatives') were making the move from health food stores to the shelves of the local supermarket. The increased availability – and diversity – of low-calorie foods fuelled the rise in snacking as cakes and cookies became, apparently, sin-free. 'Dieting is made so easy today because of the variety of low-calorie foods in the markets,' commented a still sarong-worthy Dorothy Lamour in 1956. Like millions of women in the fifties, she had discovered that she could stick to a strict calorie quota and still eat all the (diet) foods she wanted.

The 1950s was the last great era of Hollywood, as the advent of television and the subsequent arrival of the first supermodels in the 1960s soon gave women other beauties to emulate. But if the 1950s was the autumn of Hollywood's golden age, the town never shone brighter than during that last decade of supremacy. Marilyn Monroe and Audrey Hepburn became true icons who still influence both fashion and beauty standards to this day. Today, in spite of supermodels and the size-zero debate, many women still count the hourglass figure as the most attractive shape for a woman. Of course, some less positive legacies of the 1950s have been equally durable.

DIET PILLS: TAKE TWO

Originally marketed as a treatment for mild depression, during the Second World War amphetamines were widely given to soldiers – British and American; German and Japanese – as part of their general medical supplies. An unforeseen, and potentially lucrative, side effect was loss of appetite. (Other side effects included hallucinations, paranoia, mood swings, increased heart rate, strokes and tremors.)

The manufacturers soon realised that they were onto a good thing and began marketing amphetamines as weight-loss drugs. By the mid-1950s, the market was flooded with colourful copycat pills, often containing other 'goodies' like barbiturates and sedatives as well as, inevitably, a touch of metabolism-boosting thyroid hormone.

The pills were readily available on prescription and manufacturers recommended popping one or two as a preventative measure – to drop those few pounds before they became ten or twenty. Scare tactics, as ever, were omnipresent in fifties advertising. Inevitably, perfectly fit and healthy young women began queuing up to buy Obedrin, Dexamyl or AmPlus (with conveniently added vitamins).

The implication that appetite – not metabolism – was to blame for weight gain reinforced the idea (far from new, as we have seen) that whether a person was fat or thin was simply a matter of self-control. Thus to be overweight was not just unattractive but also embarrassing. You were probably eating on the sly, raiding the icebox at night when no one was there to make you feel ashamed of yourself. Is it any wonder that women – and men too – turned with relief to these supposed wonder drugs?

Unfortunately, although many of the drugs were, at least temporarily, effective, they were also found to be dangerous and highly addictive. Over the years one diet pill after another was pulled from the market, but many of them hung around until the 1970s. Today, amphetamine-based pills are completely banned in most Western countries but, worryingly, some readily-available diet pills also contain similar substances – and they can have similar side effects. What's more, amphetamine-based pills can be easily purchased online – mostly coming from South America and the Philippines – and people are buying them in their millions. You'd think we would have learned.

DIET LIKE IT'S 1955

For those who preferred not to drug themselves, the 1950s offered a smorgasbord of weight-loss plans to the determined dieter.

The Cabbage Soup Diet: This hugely popular seven-day diet consisted almost entirely of – you guessed it – cabbage soup. Other permissible foods included vegetables, fruit, skimmed milk, low-fat yoghurt, tea and coffee. The dieter might add bananas on day four, lean meat and brown rice by day six. This one came around again in the eighties and still has its advocates amongst Hollywood A-Listers today.

The Famous Clinic Diet: Remember the 'dangerous', low-calorie Hollywood Diet? It's back again under a new name. Since the experts at the Mayo Clinic were still refusing to accept responsibility, this time around *Pageant* magazine's Darlene Geis alludes simply to 'top doctors' at a 'famed medical clinic' who apparently devised the plan. Once again, the regime consists of small portions of protein with half a grapefruit to start. Except for Melba toast, carbohydrates are completely banned and coffee and other stimulants are frowned upon.

The Tapeworm Diet: A persistent urban myth, this supposed diet involves two pills: one introduces a tapeworm into the system to absorb unwanted calories; a second kills off the parasite once weight loss has been achieved. Ads for the pills existed, but whether they contained worms is another matter.

Pray Your Weight Away: Overeating had long been allied with gluttony but, in the 1950s, the connection between fat and sin was underlined by a number of diets directly targeting Christians. Reverend Charlie Shedd's 1957 bestseller *Pray Your Weight Away*, for example, recommended chanting extracts from the scriptures during exercise to help overcome the 'character flaws' that made you fat in the first place. Although the idea sounds a little kooky, it is really based on the widely accepted theory that, in some cases, weight gain may actually be psychosomatic – the link between stress and weight gain, for example, is pretty widely acknowledged. As to whether God himself is intervening on the dieter's behalf, that's another argument entirely. Whatever the truth of the matter, the Christian diet industry is still going strong today.

THE LOW-CAL REVOLUTION

'So you're on a diet? Well cheer up, fatso;
it was a lot worse twenty years ago. These days,
you can have your cake – and eat it too.'

– The Calgary Herald, 1956

The 1950s offered an array of fad diets, diet aids, weight-loss drugs and appetite suppressants – but none of these came close to matching the impact that low-calorie foods would have on the future of dieting, health and nutrition.

Holding the tantalising promise of weight loss without diet, exercise *or drugs*, low-calorie foods took off in a big way in the post-war period – especially in the USA. Including such delectable offerings as diet chocolate pudding, diet bread, sugar-free gum and even diet borscht, an ever-expanding range became readily available in supermarkets as the 1950s wore on.

You could eat them for breakfast, lunch and dinner. You didn't even have to eat separately from the rest of your family. Gone were the days of lingering mournfully over half a grapefruit as everyone else tucked into a hearty roast dinner. After all, these days you could get both the regular and diet options pre-packed and ready to go –

'A supermarket – or any kind of market – without a special diet shelf is a rarity.'

*– Garven Hudgins,
The St Petersburg Times, 1953*

how difficult was it to open a can of dietetic gravy for yourself? And as one health food manufacturer pointed out, dietetic bread was a wonderful substitute for potatoes. Sort of.

Between 1950 and 1955, sales of diet foods, sugar substitutes and diet drinks in the US increased three thousand fold and, by 1961, 40 percent of Americans were buying them. You could even get a low-cal menu on the train. And even Mrs Eisenhower reportedly bought diet items to make Ike's dinner. The low-cal revolution was slightly slower in coming to Europe, where in many places rationing continued into the fifties, but it wasn't far behind.

At a time when self-indulgence was sinful – an idea that still plagues us – low-calorie foods were apparently 'guilt free'. The lessening of the burden of guilt was undoubtedly a good thing but, on the other hand, low-cal foods also absolved any need to exercise good old self-restraint. Why practice moderation when you can have your cake and keep your figure?

Low-calorie alternatives did have their downside, of course. For one thing, they were more expensive, forcing the shopper to question whether losing an extra ten calories was actually worth another 25 cents. Catching on to the fact that they could charge more for diet items, many manufacturers simply packaged up smaller portions in order to claim a smaller calorie count – low-calorie bread, nine times out of ten, was just regular bread cut in thinner slices – it's a trick the food industry is still playing today. In future decades, people would begin to question whether sugar and fat weren't actually better for you than some of the sweeteners and low-calorie substitutes that replaced them but, for the time being, this was progress. And, in the atomic age, progress was everything.

> 'At one time a badge of shame, hallmark of the lazy lady and the careless wife, today the can opener is fast becoming a magic wand, especially in the hands of those brave, young women, nine million of them (give or take a few thousand here and there), who are engaged in frying as well as bringing home the bacon.'
>
> *– Poppy Cannon,*
> *The Can-Opener Cookbook, 1951*

> 'It's simple arithmetic. When you reduce your calories, you automatically reduce your weight. It's the calories that count. Not the amount of food that you eat, but the number of calories in it.'
>
> *– Advertisement for Tasti-Diet diet foods*

ELEVENSES WITH
Grace Kelly

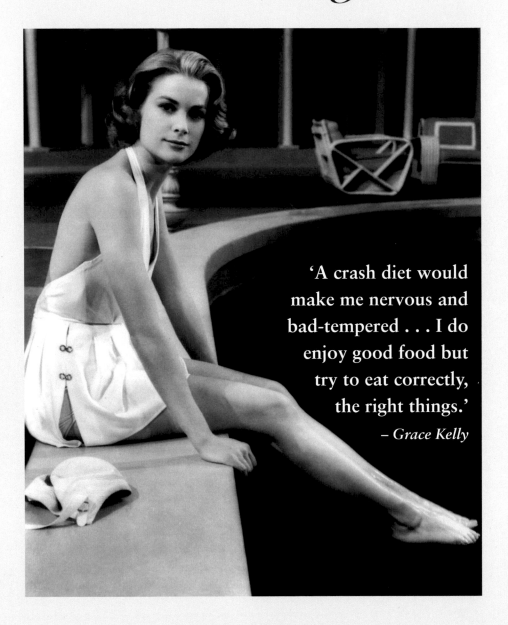

'A crash diet would make me nervous and bad-tempered . . . I do enjoy good food but try to eat correctly, the right things.'

– *Grace Kelly*

> 'My mother is German and you know
> how the Germans love to eat. We all grew up with
> pretty healthy appetites.'
>
> – *Grace Kelly*

The epitome of beauty and elegance, Grace Kelly was the Queen of Hollywood long before she became Princess of Monaco. But even Princess Grace had her flaws: at 5'6½", she was too tall for 1950s perfection and, according to famous costume designer Edith Head, she was 'too short-waisted and long-legged'. Like many of us, Grace also struggled to keep her weight under control, especially when her busy life made both eating well and exercising a challenge.

Although she came from a sport-obsessed family, when she was working, Grace rarely had time to exercise. Instead, she tackled weight gain largely through diet. For a while she followed a regime of yoghurt, yoga and berries, prescribed for her by Gayelord Hauser, but, although she was fond of all of these things, she disliked fads, preferring to stick to small portions of her usual meals. Grace had a sweet tooth and had adopted a 'just say no' policy when it came to dessert – 'I pay for it all week' – but the biggest threat to her perfect waistline was the mid-morning munchies.

Like many people who start work early, by mid-morning Grace needed a little something to keep her going until lunch. She picked up the idea of elevenses from time spent in England but, knowing how easy it is to turn to high-fat convenience foods when you're starving, she always started the day with filling oatmeal and came to set prepared with healthy nibbles like dried apricots, celery and carrot sticks.

As she got older, Grace took to yearly three-month detoxes, giving up alcohol and other stimulants in a somewhat despairing attempt to combat the rich food of Monaco. Always dignified, she also persistently refused to reveal her measurements to the gossip magazines.

> 'I have to get up at six to be at the studio on time. Oatmeal keeps me from getting hungry until eleven. If you get hungry before that, then you get started on the doughnut routine, and that can be dangerous.'
>
> – *Grace Kelly*

Jane Russell

BUILDING 'THE BODY'

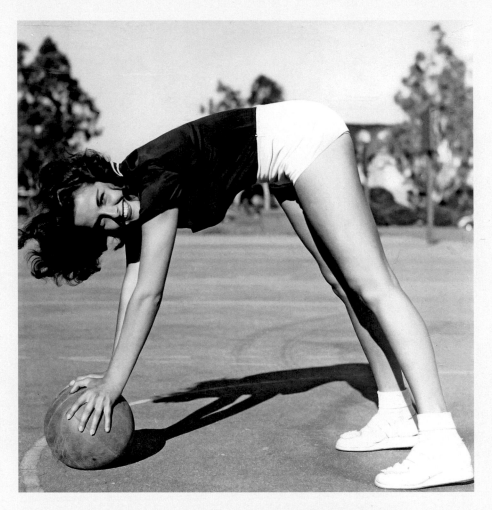

'If I skip the social cocktails I can eat
normally without bulging consequences.'

– Jane Russell

> '**My weight goes up and down and I try to catch it before it goes up more than two and a half pounds.**'
>
> – *Jane Russell*

In 1956, *The Palm Beach Daily News* predicted that, by the year 2000, the average American woman between the ages of 25 and 30 would have a figure akin to that of Jane Russell. Sadly, this hasn't come to pass. While average heights and weights have certainly increased, most women's bodies today have also lost the definition that made Jane's figure one of the most famous in history. Recent studies show that, while most women still consider the hourglass to be the most attractive figure, only a minute number still have it. Today's norm is a waistless 'apple' or 'rectangle' shape.

If we can't have Jane's figure, we can at least benefit from her attitude to weight loss, which was no-nonsense and, for a woman who spent her life being photographed, remarkably sane. Jane hated the gym and could never be bothered to count calories; if she wanted to reduce her calorie intake, she cut out beer. As for exercise, her motto was: make it fun, or you won't do it. It's a philosophy more people struggling to lose weight would do well to adopt.

JANE'S FUN SLIMMING EXERCISES

For the Waist: Hula hoop. Spinning a bamboo hoop helped Jane tighten that lovely waist.

For the Bust: Archery. Jane's favourite sport provided a full upper-body workout, keeping her famous bustline high and firm. Archery is also great for your posture; you can't expect to hit the target if you slump!

For All-Over Fitness: Outdoor sport. Jane loved swimming and skiing, tennis and golf, so it wasn't a chore for her to pick up a racket and play off the pounds. She firmly believed that every girl should take up at least one sport.

For Grace and Suppleness: Dancing – it uses all the muscles. Jane explains: 'Dancing tells a story, and to make the story smooth, one movement must flow into another and that way you move your whole body.'

Indra Devi

FIRST LADY OF YOGA

'"Yoga? No, thank you!" is what I often
heard in 1947, when I first came to America.'

– Indra Devi

In 1953, Oregon daily newspaper *The Bend Bulletin* published an article on one of Hollywood's 'sideline "stars"'. Indra Devi, said the reporter, scathingly, 'teaches movie stars to eat moss and potato water, stand on their heads, cut down on romance and tie their legs in knots. This discomfort, to some people, is known as yoga.' The people of Oregon must have had a good chuckle over the article. Surely such a crazy Californian fad would never catch on?

A Russian émigré-turned-Bollywood actress-turned yogini, Indra Devi arrived in Hollywood in 1947 to set up America's first yoga studio. Despite her critics – some of whom suspected yoga was a sex cult – Indra's studio soon became a popular haunt for many Hollywood stars who discovered that the ancient art could help them to relax, breathe better, feel better and so work better. Famous clients included Gloria Swanson, Greta Garbo, Jennifer Jones, and Marilyn Monroe. Swanson, in particular, became a close friend and was active in promoting Indra and her work.

Although she had studied in India with the legendary yoga guru Sri Tirumalai Krishnamacharya – one of the first women, let alone *Western* women to do so – Indra always stressed her identity as a Westerner, just like her students. She promoted yoga as a means to good health rather than, necessarily, to self-realisation and was careful not to push the spiritual aspect too far for her audience.

In her first book, *Forever Young, Forever Healthy*, Indra explains that there are many forms of yoga to suit different types of person, from those who wish to improve their health and figure to those seeking 'a union with the higher self'. Indra taught Hatha Yoga: 'the yoga of physical

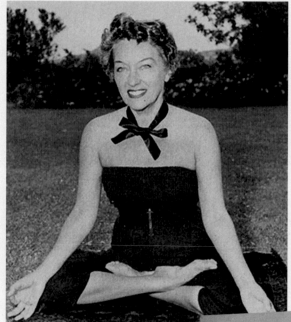

'People in most of the cases like to copy tastes and habits of their idols, thus a large number of people started to practice yoga only because [of] Gloria Swanson.'

– Indra Devi

*Above and right: **Yoga's First Lady, Indra Devi**, practices with pupil and friend Gloria Swanson. The images feature in Devi's second book,* Yoga for Americans *(1948).*

perfection'. (No wonder it was popular in Hollywood.) Besides improving their health, Indra promised that yoga would help her students to shed excess weight, clear the complexion, and roll back the clock on wrinkles.

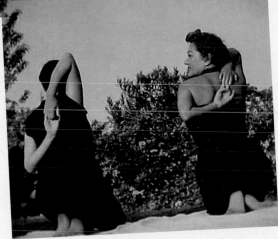

'A person who learns to relax learns the secret of a successful and healthy, long life.'

– Indra Devi

Marilyn Monroe

FITNESS TRAILBLAZER

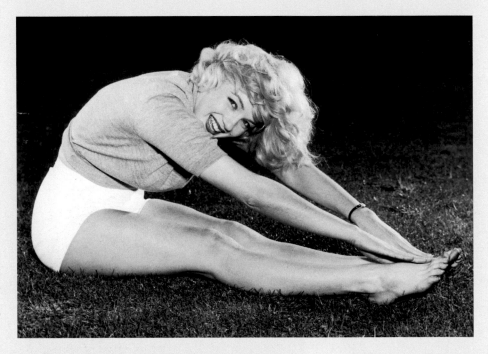

'I spend at least ten minutes each morning working out with small weights. I have evolved my own exercises for the muscles I wish to keep firm, and I know they are right for me because I can feel them putting the proper muscles into play as I exercise.'

– *Marilyn Monroe*

'I couldn't stand exercise if I had to feel regimented about it.'

– Marilyn Monroe

Years after Jean Harlow vacated Hollywood's throne, there was a new platinum blonde in town. Destined to outshine even her idol, Marilyn Monroe would become one of the most iconic actresses ever to emerge from the movies.

Almost an exaggeration of the fifties ideal, Marilyn combined sex appeal with unthreatening, little-girlish femininity. Studios dressed her in a way that left little to the imagination. The sumptuous silks and daring cut of her costumes were designed not to inhibit the view of what lay beneath. Marilyn rarely wore a corset (or indeed, any underwear at all). Her figure didn't need much help and, besides, her outfits were so tight, she often had to be sewn into them.

In Marilyn's view every girl should free herself from the tyranny of corsets. Well, almost every girl: 'First, some of them ought to exercise to be . . . you know . . . firm,' she added cautiously. Of course, she was only offering the advice she followed herself. Marilyn took the task of maintaining her body very seriously and, alongside traditional 'ladies' exercises', like swimming, tennis and calisthenics, her daily routine using light weights appears surprisingly modern.

Unlike many actresses of the day, Marilyn did not simply go through the motions of exercising, slavishly following a plan laid out by the studio fitness guru. Instead, she worked out her own routine, paying close attention to which muscles she was using and to how they felt when she moved. Influenced by Mabel Elsworth Todd's 1937 work, *The Thinking Body*, Marilyn was keen to understand the way the individual parts – nerves, muscles, bones – worked as a unit to create a certain outward appearance and how the body might be taught to assume new ways of standing, moving and reacting. Marilyn believed strongly in the connection between mind, movement, self-improvement and posture: ideas that led her to the practice of yoga.

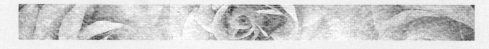

MARILYN THE YOGI

Working with Indra Devi, Marilyn Monroe was one of several film stars who took up yoga years before this flexibility-enhancing trend caught on in the rest of the Western world. Regular practice would have tightened her waist, leaving curves in all the right places.

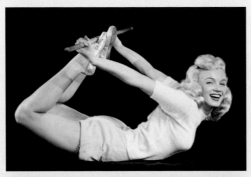

1. BOW POSE

This pose expands the chest, improves posture and strengthens back muscles. It also relieves anxiety and fatigue and aids digestion.

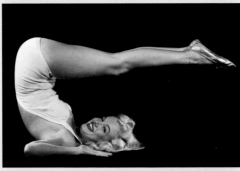

2. PLOW POSE

This pose stretches the spine and tones the shoulders, hamstrings, and abdomen. The position also triggers the release of endorphins, relieving pain and stress.

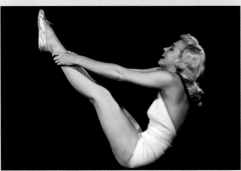

3. BOAT POSE

This pose improves balance, calms the mind, and relieves stress – all whilst toning the abdominal muscles.

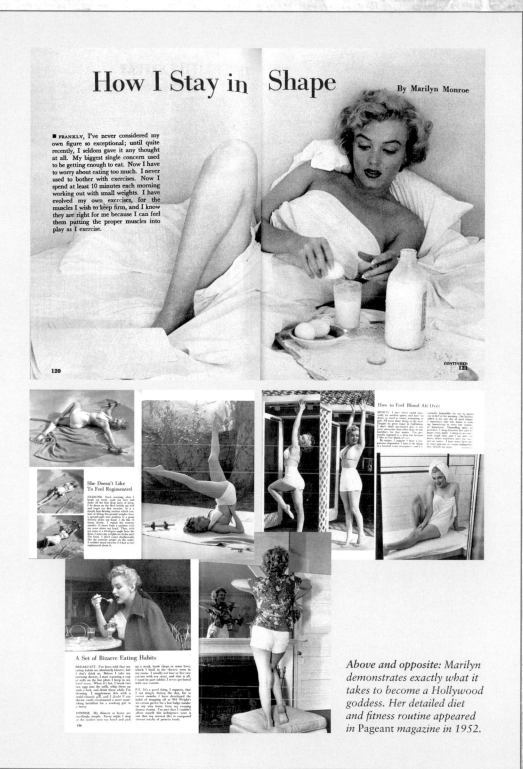

Above and opposite: Marilyn demonstrates exactly what it takes to become a Hollywood goddess. Her detailed diet and fitness routine appeared in Pageant magazine in 1952.

MARILYN'S MENU

'Frankly, I've never considered my figure so exceptional. My biggest single concern used to be getting enough to eat.'

– Marilyn Monroe

Although she usually skipped lunch, thought ice cream sundaes were an acceptable meal substitute, and risked salmonella poisoning every morning with her warm milk and raw egg combo, Marilyn's diet was less extreme than those practiced by many stars of the day. What's more, it was recommended by a doctor (unlike, for example, the aspirin-and-coffee plan once employed by Betty Hutton). Although Marilyn's menu is protein-heavy, the meat she chooses is lean and her favourite, liver, is especially rich in nutrients. Her shopping lists show that, when she wasn't filming, her diet was actually reasonably varied and, unlike her idol Jean Harlow, she never seems to have binged between movies.

Breakfast: Two raw eggs mixed in hot milk (sometimes with sherry, if she was feeling under the weather). One multivitamin pill. 'I doubt if any doctor could prescribe a more nourishing breakfast for a working girl in a hurry.'

Dinner: High-nutrient meat – typically lamb chops, steak, or liver – roasted in the oven, with four or five raw carrots on the side. 'My dinners at home are startlingly simple.'

On Her Shopping List: Artichokes, eggs, English muffins, cucumber, radishes, strawberry jam, cheddar cheese, corn-on-the-cob, strawberries, endives, steaks, milk, lamb chops, and chicken.

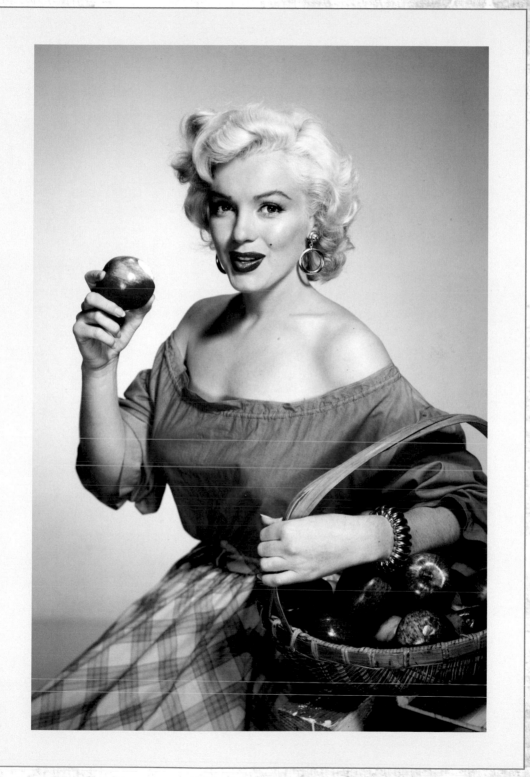

Jack LaLanne

THE GODFATHER OF FITNESS

'Exercise is king. Nutrition is queen.
Put them together and you've got a kingdom!'

– Jack LaLanne

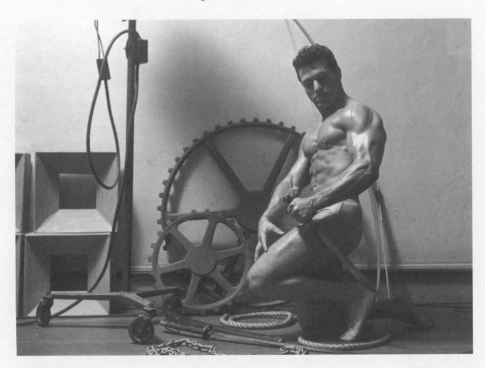

Jack LaLanne is rightly remembered as the godfather of modern fitness. He set up the world's first modern health club in Oakland, California in 1936; it grew to a chain of over 200 centres. He promoted weight training for women and athletes at a time when neither group lifted. Women were told they would turn into men; athletes would become slow and muscle-bound. He contended that elderly people not only could but *should* exercise regularly – an idea not then supported by America's doctors. He also invented a lot of the equipment you're probably familiar with from your local gym, like leg-extension machines and weight selectors.

In the 1950s, LaLanne used America's first nationally syndicated TV fitness show to encourage ordinary people to work out. Household objects – a chair or a broom – provided all the necessary equipment and you could do the routines in your own living room. The show ran for 34 years, earning LaLanne millions of fans – Hollywood's finest amongst them – and his own star on the Hollywood walk of fame.

JACK LALANNE'S 10 POINT SELF-IMPROVEMENT PLAN

'Today we're trying to think of improvement, students, not only the physical part – you having a nicer figure – but we're thinking about the spiritual aspect and the mental aspect of it.'

1. Exercise: 'If you don't exercise, you're going to look and feel old.'

2. Nutrition: 'You're intelligent; you know the foods you shouldn't be eating.'

3. Positive Thinking: 'Appreciate what you have and don't be thinking about the things that you don't have.'

4. Good Habits: 'Start replacing some of your bad habits with good habits.'

5. Grooming: 'Some of you girls get in a rut: you don't fix your hair as good as you used to and your clothes are not quite as neat as they used to be . . . Make you a lovelier you so you can start getting compliments from the man in your life.'

6. Smile: 'A smile is infectious: you'll have other people liking you more and you'll be enjoying yourself more.'

7. Posture: 'Pull that old tummy and shoulders back!'

8. Help Others: 'Pass the word around about this little get together, about our philosophy of living, about correct exercise and nutrition.'

9. Relaxation: 'Spare five or ten minutes to lie down in a dark room, completely relaxed, if you can sleep so much the better. That helps to release all this nervous tension and build up this old energy and vitality that we need.'

10. Faith: 'If you make an effort to do these things, God helps those who help themselves.'

Audrey Hepburn's
MENU

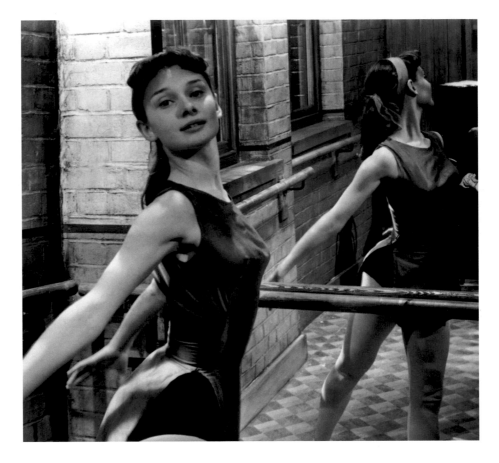

'Even if you don't intend to make a career out of ballet, the training develops grace, equilibrium and freedom and clarity of movement.'

– *Audrey Hepburn*

'After so many drive-in waitresses becoming movie stars, there has been this real drought, when along comes class; somebody who actually went to school, can spell, maybe even plays the piano.'

– Billy Wilder

When Audrey Hepburn first arrived in Hollywood, the prevailing fashion was for curvy sweater girls. But as Audrey herself famously said, 'There is more to sex appeal than just measurements.' As she skyrocketed to stardom, her waif-like figure foreshadowed the coming sixties trend. Today, Audrey is one of the most imitated women of all time, the epitome of charm and effortless chic.

Audrey's girlish physique was based on years of ballet – and an undernourished childhood in occupied Holland. Never having been used to large meals growing up, she never developed much of an appetite. Her very slender figure has led some people to suggest that Audrey was anorexic, but, according to her friends and family, this simply wasn't true. In fact, after starving for much of her childhood, it would also have gone against the grain with her to starve herself voluntarily. Like many children of the Second World War, Audrey had a huge respect for food and hated waste. She was a firm believer in eating well and getting enough nutrients. To her, this meant 'three full meals a day with at least one serving of red meat' and, when necessary, vitamin supplements.

'I seem to have a sort of built-in leveller. I've a tremendously good appetite – I eat everything, everything – but as soon as I'm satisfied a little hatch closes up and I stop.'

– Audrey Hepburn

Audrey was introduced to supplements by fashionable nutritionist, Adelle Davis, who showed her how the right ones could make a huge difference to her wellbeing. Audrey took her suggestions to heart and, like many people at this time, consumed an array of vitamins every day, her favourites being Vitamin A to combat fatigue and 'the anti-infection vitamin', Vitamin C.

> **'When I look at something such as a white slice of sugary cake, I have no desire for it because I know it will do nothing at all for me.'**
>
> *– Audrey Hepburn*

Audrey was 'not a snacker' and she didn't believe in indulging or swallowing empty calories. Her one weakness was chocolates but, with strong self-discipline, she never allowed her fondness to become a problem, saying simply, 'If I ate all I wanted it just wouldn't do.' Although many of us would struggle to maintain a healthy weight on Audrey's austere menu, there is a lot we can learn from her post-war attitude to food. Not only did Audrey respect her body by only putting into it food she considered healthy, her thrifty attitude ensured she did not waste food either: her eyes were *never* bigger than her stomach and her waist was tiny.

AUDREY'S AUSTERE MENU

Breakfast: Two boiled eggs; one slice seven-grain, whole-wheat toast; three to four cups coffee with hot milk.

Lunch: Cottage cheese with fruit or yoghurt followed by raw vegetables.

Dinner: Red meat with several cooked vegetables or pasta and salad. Occasionally, a glass of wine.

Supplements: On the advice of fashionable nutritionist Adelle Davis, Audrey supplemented her meals with daily vitamins: **Vitamin A** to combat fatigue; **Vitamin C** to fight infection; and **Powdered Liver** taken in a cup of consommé whenever she needed an energy boost.

Audrey's Top Tip: Sit up straight! 'Nothing is worse for the waistline than slumping.'

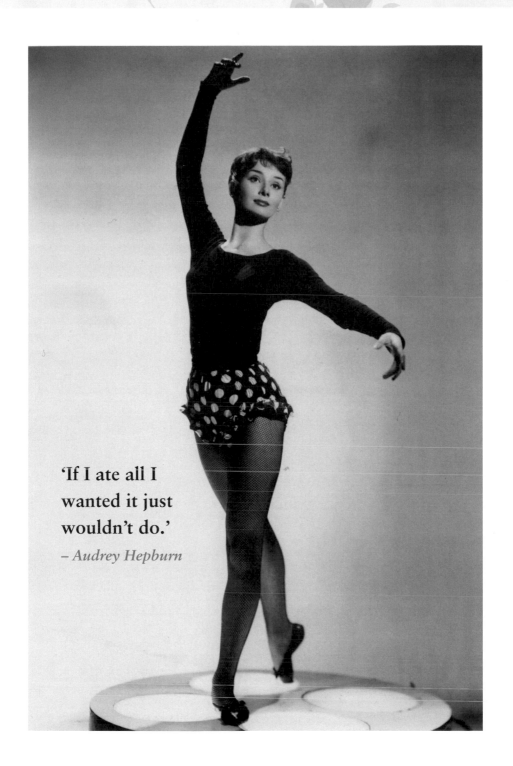

'If I ate all I
wanted it just
wouldn't do.'
– *Audrey Hepburn*

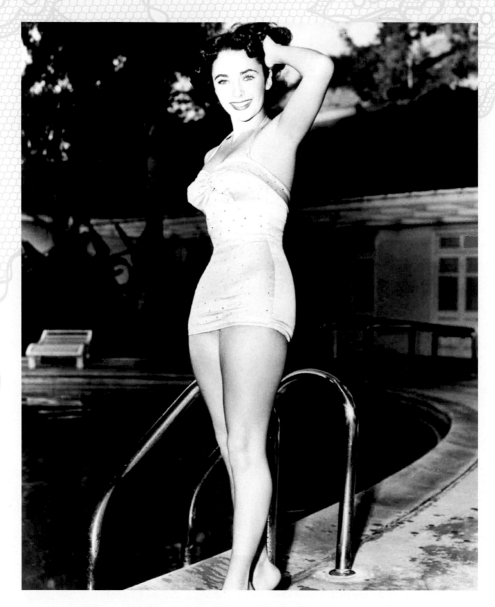

'The problem with people who have no vices
is that you can be sure they're going to have
some pretty annoying virtues.'

– *Elizabeth Taylor*

AFTERWORD

The Resistance

'I do everything they say you shouldn't.
I eat and drink what I like. I stay up late.'

– Ingrid Bergman

In the Golden Age of Hollywood, actresses worked hard – or so they were keen to impress upon their public. 'Think you'd like to be a movie star? Think again!' they told fans, shaking their beautiful heads at such naivety. You have to be in makeup at six in the morning, memorise a whole bunch of lines, work all hours. You'd be too exhausted to go out on the town, and when you *did* show up at a function or premiere you would have to appear flawless. Naturally, you'd have a strict exercise routine and an even stricter diet. You'd never eat a dessert again. That's just what it takes to be a star.

Some stars, however, didn't get the memo. Even in the world of movies, where those two extra pounds look like ten, there were girls who ate (and drank) what they liked, heedless of the consequences. I don't mean the emaciated starlets who swore they never stinted themselves but ran a mile from a dish of mashed potatoes or spoonful of rich chocolate mousse. I mean the likes of Elizabeth Taylor, who declared proudly, 'I'm willing to be stuck with what God gave me' – and meant it.

Of course, most of us would be happy with what God gave Liz. In spite of a daily diet calculated to add pounds and clog arteries, she was repeatedly hailed as the most beautiful girl in movies. She must have had very good genes to eat so much bacon and peanut butter – along with generous helpings of alcohol – and still keep that figure for so many years.

In her forties, Liz *did* begin to struggle with her weight, ballooning up to 180 lbs before finally succumbing to a diet of her own devising. She regained her ideal weight of 120 lbs using a regime that included

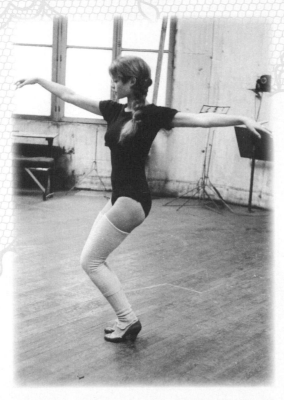

'My favourite sport is cha-cha-cha.'

– Brigitte Bardot

recipes such as cottage cheese mixed with sour cream, 'pig out days' once a week, and some very half-hearted exercise routines. Liz shared the diet in a book called *Elizabeth Takes Off*. The fact that it became a bestseller surely has more to do with the magnetism of Elizabeth Taylor than the diet plan itself.

On the other side of the Atlantic, the sex kitten of the French movie scene, Brigitte Bardot, was similarly uninterested in the healthy lifestyle expected of a star. BB's astonishing 36-19-36 figure was founded on years of ballet – she trained for two hours a day from the age of seven until her late teens – but maintained with no more effort than it took to pout. 'I'm very fortunate to have my shape, I know,' she shrugged, 'but that's the way it is.'

Brigitte was 'not the sporty type', she practiced no regular exercise and never swallowed a vitamin pill in her life. She ate whatever she wanted – from a cheese-laden croque-monsieur to spaghetti with a (large) glass of red wine – and though later in life she would become a vegetarian, for ethical reasons, she never dieted. At the age of 40, having retired from the screen to focus on 'life', she was still confident enough in her figure to pose naked for playboy.

The true queen of the anti-dieters, however, is Ingrid Bergman, who had a normal, healthy figure and resisted the collective urging of her director, the critics and her first husband, Peter Lindstrom, to change this. Although she once sighed that everybody would have been happier if she just weighed five pounds less, Ingrid never stinted herself, her

> ## 'I even dreamed about ice cream. Those were good dreams.'
> *– Ingrid Bergman*

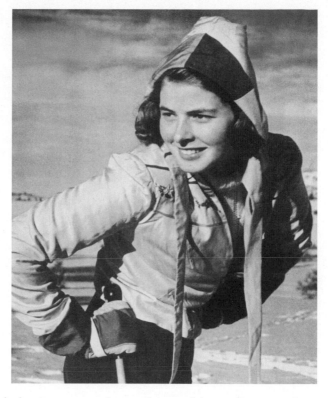

only exercise was of the hearty, outdoor kind, 'like everybody else in Sweden', and her only beauty secret was being Ingrid Bergman . . . and ice cream.

Ingrid considered American ice cream – so much creamier than in Europe – to be an 'unbelievable delight' and, in New York, where she liked the ice cream best, she could eat four sundaes in one day, going to different parlours to avoid embarrassment. In the evening, she switched to another American speciality: cocktails. 'When I came to America and saw all the names – stingers, daiquiris – I just started with "A" and went down the list,' she said simply. Ingrid remained contentedly a few pounds over what Hollywood considered ideal for her entire career: the public loved her.

Today, the pressure on young actresses to conform to unrealistic standards of beauty is still strong – witness Jennifer Lawrence, who has been applauded for saying she'd rather look chubby on screen and 'like a person' in real life. Celebrities' exercise routines, real and suspected diets, and struggles with extra pounds continue to feature heavily in tabloids and magazines. And the figures we see on the big (and now small) screen continue to influence our ideas of what is desirable. Surely there's something we can learn from these girls, who took life as it came and were happy in their own skins – even if there's not a nutritionist alive who would recommend their diet choices!

British Library Cataloguing in Publication Data
A catalogue record for this book is available from
the British Library

ISBN-13: 978-0-85965-502-6

Cover photos by John Kobal Foundation/Moviepix/
Getty Images and Movie Market
Cover and book design by Coco Wake-Porter
Printed in China on behalf of Latitude Press Ltd
by WKT Company Ltd

BIBLIOGRAPHY

Books: *Greta Garbo: A Life Apart*, Karen Swenson; *Garbo*,
Barry Paris; *Notorious: The Life of Ingrid Bergman*, Donald Spoto;
Ingrid: A Personal Biography, Charlotte Chandler; *Ava Gardner:
Love is Nothing*, Lee Server; *Fat History: Bodies and Beauty in
the Modern West*, Peter N. Stearns; *No Food with My Meals*,
Fanny Hurst; *Health via Food*, William Howard Hay; *Calories
and Corsets: A History of Dieting Over Two Thousand Years*,
Louise Foxcroft; *The Fixers: Eddie Mannix, Howard Strickling and
the MGM Publicity Machine*, E.J. Fleming; *Obesity: A Reference
Handbook*, Judith S. Stern, Alexandra Kazaks; *Diet and Health:
With Key to the Calories*, Lulu Hunt Peters; *Hollywood Goes
Shopping*, David Desser; *Hollywood and the Rise of Physical
Culture*, Heather Addison; *How to be Lovely: The Audrey Hepburn
Way of Life*, Melissa Hellstern; *Food is Your Best Medicine*, Dr
Henry Bieler; *History of Meals for Millions, Soy, and Freedom from
Hunger: Extensively Annotated Bibliography and Sourcebook*,
William Shurtleff; *Marlene Dietrich's ABC*, Marlene Dietrich; *Dr
Atkins New Diet Revolution*, Robert C. Atkins; *How to Always
Be Well*, William Howard Hay; *The Hay Diet Made Easy*, Jackie
Habgood; *Food Combining Diet: The Healthy Way to Lose Weight*,
Kathryn Marsden; *The Hungry Years: Confessions of a Food
Addict*, William Leith; *The Hundred Year Diet: America's Voracious
Appetite for Losing Weight*, Susan Yager; *The Dukan Diet*, Dr
Pierre Dukan; *Mrs Richter's Cook-Less Book*, Vera M. Richter;
Forever Young, Forever Healthy, Indra Devi; *Yoga For Americans*,
Indra Devi; *Pull Yourself Together, Baby*, Sylvia Ullback; *Hollywood
Undressed: Observations of Sylvia As Noted by Her Secretary*,
Sylvia Ullback; *No More Alibis*, Sylvia Ullback.

Magazines and newspapers: *Photoplay*, *Physical Culture*,
Motion Picture Magazine, *Motion Picture Classic*, *Picturegoer*,
Radio Mirror, *Spot* magazine, *Pageant* magazine, *Youngstown
Vindicator*, *Evening Independent*, *Milwaukee Sentinel*, *Sydney
Morning Herald*, *The Meridian Daily Journal*, *Milwaukee Journal*,
Ottawa Citizen, *Ocala Star Banner*, *Los Angeles Times*, *The Palm
Beach Post*, *The Virgin Islands Daily News*, *The Miami News*,
Pittsburgh Post-Gazette, *The Spokesman Review*, *The Pittsburgh
Press*, *Rochester Journal*, *Rochester Evening Journal*, *Literary
Digest*, *Daily Boston Globe*, *New York Times*, *The Bend Bulletin*,
The Florence Times Daily, *Toledo Blade*, *Gadsden Times*, *Chicago
Daily Tribune*, *The Victoria Advocate*, *The Montreal Gazette*, *The
Calgary Herald*, *The Daily Times*, *The Dispatch*, *The Baltimore
Sun*, *Long Island Star Journal*, *The Vancouver Sun*, *Daytona Beach
Sunday News Journal*, *Palm Bach Post*, *Utica Daily Press*, *Reading
Eagle*, *The Spokane Review*, *Warsaw Union*, *Ellensburg Daily
Record*, *The Hartford Courant*, *St. Petersburg Times*, *Berkeley Daily
Gazette*, *Sarasota Herald-Tribune*, *Deseret News*, *Record-Tribune
& Winnett Times*, *The Robesonian*, *Youngstown Vindicator*, *The
Telegraph-Herald and Times-Journal*, *Lewiston Evening Journal*,
The Toledo News Bee, *Toledo Blade*, *Prescott Evening Courier*,
Williamson Daily News, *Berkeley Daily Gazette*, *St. Joseph News-
Press*, *Eugene Register Guard*, *The Lewiston Daily Sun*, *Oxnard
Press-Courier*, *The Free Lance-Star*, *Star News*, *Lawrence Journal
World*, *Warsaw Times Union*, *Harper's Bazaar*, *Slate*, *The Daily
Mail*, *The Daily Telegraph*, *Vanity Fair*, *LIFE*, *People*.

Journals: 'World War II and Fashion: The Birth of the New
Look,' Lauren Olds, *Constructing the Past*, 2001; 2:47-64;
'Cookery and Digestibility,' *Journal of the American Medical
Association*, 1931; 96(24):2038-2039; 'Oracles of the New Age',
Yoga Journal, 1980 Jan-Feb; 30:9; 'The Grand Dame of Yoga',
Audrey Youngman, *Yoga Journal*, 1996 Oct; 130:74; 'America's
First Amphetamine Epidemic 1929-1971: A Quantitative and
Qualitative Retrospective With Implications for the Present',
Nicolas Rasmussen, PhD, MPhil, MPH, *Am J Public Health*, 2008
June; 98(6):974-985; 'Similar weight loss with low-energy food
combining or balanced diets,' A. Golay, A.F. Allaz, J. Ybarra,
P. Bianchi, S. Saraiva, N. Mensi, R. Gomis and N. de Tonnac,
Int J Obes Relat Metab Disord, 2000 Apr; 24(4):492-6.

Websites: dailymail.co.uk, shape.com, dietsinreview.com,
csusmhistory.org, news.bbc.co.uk, newstatesman.com, nymag.com/
thecut, www.nytimes.com, www.famous-women-and-beauty.com,
www.modernmom.com, today.msnbc.msn.com,
Stealtheirstyle.co.uk, www.xtimeline.com, www.garboforever.com,
www.ivu.org, www.arnoldehret.org, www.cbsnews.com,
www.people.com, www.msnbc.msn.com, www.historyextra.com,
www.utexas.edu/opa/blogs/culturalcompass,
www.soilandhealth.org, www.diet.com, www.netfit.co.uk,
museum.nist.gov, Everdayhealth.com, guestofaguest.com,
weightlossresources.com, Acefitness.com, www.independent.co.uk,
www.medicalnewstoday.com, blogs.lt.vt.edu/odie663,
www.drfuhrman.com, www.bda.uk.com, theyogablog.com,
amazingwomeninhistory.com, yogajournal.com,
www.livestrong.com, www.health.com, www.theday.com,
www.webmd.com, www.whfoods.com, historiful.tumblr.com,
glamourmagazine.co.uk, www.jacklalanne.com, www.halls.md,
www.oprah.com, www.thedietchanel.com, www.wewomen.com,
www.second-opinions.co.uk, www.accesshollywood.com,
uk.atkins.com, thisrecording.com, content.time.com, people.com,
zumba.com, www.mirror.co.uk.

Radio: *Svelte Sylvia and the Hollywood Trimsters*, Karen
Krizanovich, BBC Radio 4.

We would also like to thank the following for supplying
photographs: Virgil Apger/John Kobal Foundation/Moviepix/
Getty Images; Eugene Robert Richee/John Kobal Foundation/
Moviepix/Getty Images; Movie Market; Ernest Bachrach/John
Kobal Foundation/Moviepix/Getty Images; Max Munn Autrey/
Stringer/General Photographic Agency/Moviepix/Getty Images;
Alfred Eisenstaedt/Pix Inc./Time Life Pictures/Getty Images; Don
Gillum/John Kobal Foundation/Moviepix/Getty Images; General
Photographic Agency/Stringer/Hulton Archive/Getty Images; Laszlo
Willinger/John Kobal Foundation/Moviepix/Getty Images; General
Photographic Agency/Hulton Archive/Getty Images; Underwood
Archives/Archive Photos/Getty Images; Hulton Archive/Stringer/
Moviepix/Getty Images; John Kobal Foundation/Moviepix/Getty
Images; Popperfoto/Getty Images; Bernard Hoffman/Pictures Inc./
Time Life Pictures/Getty Images; Graphic House/Archive Photos/
Archive Photos/Getty Images; Eric Carpenter/John Kobal
Foundation/Moviepix/Getty Images; Dave Cicero/Stringer/ Hulton
Archive/Archive Photos/Getty Images; Nickolas Muray/George
Eastman House/Archive Photos/Getty Images; National Film
Archive London; John Sadovy/BIPs/Stringer/Hulton Archive/Getty
Images; Bob Landry/Time Life Pictures/Getty Images.